Healthcare Coverage and Disability Evaluation for Reserve Component Personnel

Research for the 11th Quadrennial Review of Military Compensation

Susan D. Hosek

Prepared for the Office of the Secretary of Defense
Approved for public release; distribution unlimited

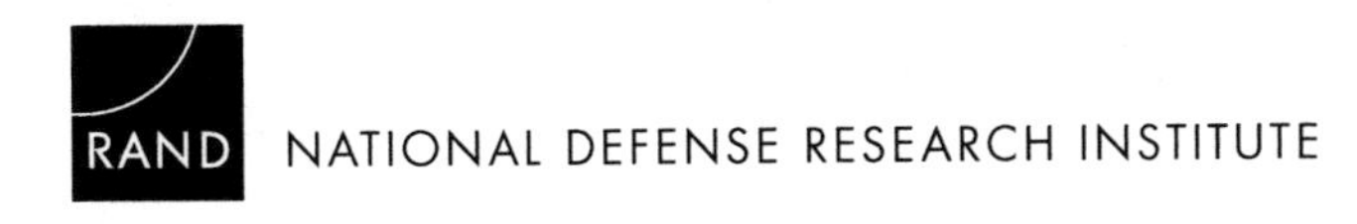

The research described in this report was prepared for the Office of the Secretary of Defense (OSD). The research was conducted within the RAND National Defense Research Institute, a federally funded research and development center sponsored by OSD, the Joint Staff, the Unified Combatant Commands, the Navy, the Marine Corps, the defense agencies, and the defense Intelligence Community under Contract W74V8H-06-C-0002.

Library of Congress Control Number: 2012942907

ISBN: 978-0-8330-5936-9

Cover: A wounded U.S. Marine walks through the halls of the U.S. military's Ibn Sina Hospital in the Green Zone of Baghdad, 2004 (AP Photo/John Moore).

Published 2012 by the RAND Corporation
1776 Main Street, P.O. Box 2138, Santa Monica, CA 90407-2138
1200 South Hayes Street, Arlington, VA 22202-5050
4570 Fifth Avenue, Suite 600, Pittsburgh, PA 15213-2665
RAND URL: http://www.rand.org/
To order RAND documents or to obtain additional information, contact
Distribution Services: Telephone: (310) 451-7002;
Fax: (310) 451-6915; Email: order@rand.org

Preface

Federal law mandates that every four years the President assess the military compensation system. The eleventh such review, known as the 11th Quadrennial Review of Military Compensation (QRMC), focuses on four broad areas. Two of these areas concern compensation and benefits for members of the Reserve Component (RC) and for wounded personnel. RC members have been increasingly used in an operational capacity, and the 11th QRMC is therefore investigating healthcare coverage and disability evaluation for those who are wounded, injured, or ill because of their military service. As part of the review, RAND was asked to analyze healthcare coverage for RC members, including participation in the TRICARE Reserve Select (TRS) program, the potential effects of national health reform on coverage rates, and disability evaluation outcomes for RC members. This report summarizes the results of RAND's analysis. The findings should be of interest to the RC policy community as well as those interested in military health and disability issues more broadly.

The research was sponsored by the 11th QRMC and conducted within the Forces and Resources Policy Center of the RAND National Defense Research Institute, a federally funded research and development center sponsored by the Office of the Secretary of Defense, the Joint Staff, the Unified Combatant Commands, the Navy, the Marine Corps, the defense agencies, and the defense Intelligence Community. Assistance was provided by RAND Health's Center for Military Health Policy Research.

For more information on the Center for Military Health Policy Research, see http://www.rand.org/multi/military.html or contact the director (contact information is provided on the web page). For more information on the RAND Forces and Resources Policy Center, see http://www.rand.org/nsrd/ndri/centers/frp.html or contact the director (contact information is provided on the web page).

Contents

Figures

Tables

Summary

The use of Reserve Component (RC) personnel has increased dramatically since September 11, 2001, and has remained high. Both Active Component (AC) and RC personnel serving on active duty for more than 30 days have comprehensive healthcare coverage, but other RC members are covered only for injuries or illness sustained in the line of duty. For other conditions, they must rely on their civilian healthcare coverage—if they have such coverage. A decade of combat, however, has focused the nation's attention on meeting the needs of service members—both AC and RC—whose military service has led to disability.

Legislation passed in 1965 required the President to review military compensation every four years. In light of the critical role the RC has played and is likely to continue to play in the future, the President asked the 11th Quadrennial Review of Military Compensation (QRMC) to examine compensation and benefits for RC personnel. As part of this review, RAND was asked to provide supporting analyses of the healthcare coverage provided for RC members, including participation in the TRS program, the potential effects of national health reform on coverage rates, and disability evaluation outcomes for RC members.

Findings on Healthcare Coverage

To assess the rates of health insurance coverage among RC members, we relied on the Status of Forces Survey of Reserve Component Personnel (SoF-R). This survey is administered to a sample of Selected Reserve members twice a year; every two years, the survey asks respondents whether they have health/medical insurance. The most recent SoF-R, fielded in January 2011, indicated that 30 percent of Selected Reserve members lack health insurance. Uninsured members are more likely to be unemployed or to work part time or for a small firm; they are also younger and have less education than those with insurance. The percentage of uninsured in the Selected Reserve population closely mirrors the percentage in the comparable civilian population.

We obtained data on TRS enrollment from the Defense Enrollment and Eligibility Reporting System (DEERS), the official enrollment file for TRICARE, the healthcare program serving active-duty service members, National Guard and Reserve members, retirees, families, and survivors. DEERS information about members is more limited than that provided by the SoF-R, but DEERS is more current and its TRS enrollment data are more reliable. The TRS program was initiated to offer insurance for RC members who lack a civilian option, and both TRS eligibility and affordability have changed significantly in recent years. Our analysis finds that TRS enrollment grew rapidly after the changes were implemented and included 8 percent of the eligible population in June 2010. While it is possible that insurance coverage in this population has not declined because of TRS, the evidence suggests that quite a few enrollees have access to civilian insurance that they find less attractive. Further, the characteristics of TRS enrollees do not match well with the characteristics of uninsured RC members.

Although at present the TRS program may not be significantly reducing the number of uninsured RC members, this may change if an individual insurance mandate and associated penalties are implemented in 2014 in accordance with the Patient Protection and Affordable Care Act (PPACA). To gain insight into the potential effects of PPACA on health insurance coverage of RC members in the absence of TRS, we applied results from the RAND COMPARE microsimulation model of health reform to estimate the changes in the percentage of RC members with insurance and in the sources of insurance. The model predicts how individuals and firms are likely to respond to healthcare policy changes, including those in PPACA, based on the economic theory of health decisionmaking and accumulated evidence from more modest policy changes (e.g., changes in Medicaid eligibility). Our analysis finds that health reform can be expected to increase the rate of insured RC members to 89 percent. The model projects that 12 percent will be eligible for Medicaid once eligibility is expanded, and another 12 percent will purchase coverage through state-level health insurance exchanges. Four-fifths of the latter will be eligible for a subsidy.

These projections do not factor in the availability of TRS. Many RC members who would otherwise purchase coverage from the health insurance exchanges are likely to find TRS more attractive financially. The TRS costs compare favorably with those of the health insurance plans that will be offered by the state health exchanges, even for members at income levels eligible for subsidies in the exchanges. In addition, some fraction of the 11 percent of RC members predicted to remain uninsured by the COMPARE model would enroll in TRS instead. TRS premiums for single and family coverage are, at worst, only slightly higher than the penalty for having no insurance under health reform. Therefore, there is a good chance that health reform will induce a further increase in TRS enrollment. This increase would be in addition to any increase in the number of RC members enrolling in TRS instead of taking up their employer coverage and could make it very difficult to achieve the goal of controlling the health costs of the Department of Defense (DoD).

DoD is already providing healthcare coverage to a majority of working-age military retirees and will have to assume a substantial role in covering RC members as well.

In 2007, the DoD Task Force on the Future of the Military Heath System called attention to the increasing number of non–active-duty beneficiaries who choose TRICARE instead of employer benefits. The task force recommended considering a pilot program to test a benefit that would supplement rather than substitute for employer benefits. Such an initiative should include RC members in addition to retirees.

Findings on Disability Outcomes for RC Members

To examine the disposition of disability outcomes for RC members, we used data provided by the Army, Navy, and Air Force on all disability cases that were initiated in fiscal years 2007–2010 and for which an informal board decision had been made. The data capture the early effects of the important changes in the DoD and Department of Veterans Affairs (VA) disability evaluation systems that were made during that time. Our analysis finds that, as with healthcare, the major difference in disability evaluation of RC and AC members results from the line-of-duty requirement. AC members are considered to be continuously on duty, so the health problems that arise while they are in service are almost always a basis for disability benefits. RC members are not covered for disabilities that are not incurred or aggravated as a result of training or active service. Furthermore, RC members are only approximately one-third as likely to be referred to the Disability Evaluation System (DES) as AC members. Given this difference, war-related medical conditions are more common among RC members, but it is not possible to conclude from the available data whether all RC members with line-of-duty conditions are identified and evaluated for disability.

The rates of referral for post-traumatic stress disorder (PTSD) for RC and AC members who have deployed since 2001 are 1.4 per 1,000 members and 3.0 per 1,000 members, respectively. This difference is hard to understand given the evidence that the incidence of PTSD is at least as high in the RC. The identification of RC members who experience health consequences leading to disability resulting from deployment merits further investigation.

Once referred for disability evaluation, the process is the same across components, and there is little difference between RC and AC dispositions. For those with PTSD, the strict policy guidance of placement on the Temporary Disability Retirement List (TDRL) ensures equal outcomes. For others, once the medical condition captured by the Veteran Affairs Schedule of Rating Disabilities (VASRD) code is controlled for, the differences are only a few percentage points at most.

Acknowledgments

The author is indebted to a number of individuals who contributed to this study. Tom Bush, the Director of the 11th QRMC, provided helpful guidance and support throughout the research. Ron Hunter, the Deputy Director, was indefatigable in arranging for provision of the data used in the study, and he facilitated the research in a number of other ways. The disability data files were provided with the assistance of David Turban and Michael Carino for the Army, Robert Powers for the Navy, and Susan Nunnery for the Air Force. They also provided valuable information about their services' disability evaluation procedures and answered a number of questions about the data. Several RAND colleagues made important contributions to the analysis. Heather Krull developed the data used in the analysis of health reform effects and collaborated with Carter Price in producing the predicted outcomes from health reform. Craig Martin provided invaluable assistance by piecing together the disability data for the services and programming all analyses of these data. Stephanie Williamson and Arthur Bullock provided programming assistance for the analysis of the Status of Forces and DEERS data, respectively. Jake Soloman and Gail Fisher provided general research assistance, and Paul Steinberg drafted the Summary of the monograph. I wish to thank Paul Hogan and Seth Seabury for their thoughtful reviews of the draft. Finally, I appreciate the support of the leaders of the RAND project that included this research, Beth Asch and Jim Hosek.

Abbreviations

AC	Active Component
AGR	Active Guard Reserve
CPS	Current Population Survey
CRDP	Concurrent Retirement and Disability Payment
CRSC	Combat-Related Special Compensation
DEERS	Defense Enrollment and Eligibility Reporting System
DES	Disability Evaluation System
DMDC	Defense Manpower Data Center
DoD	Department of Defense
EPTS	existing prior to service
FEHB	Federal Employee Health Benefits
FPL	federal poverty level
HMO	health maintenance organization
IDES	Integrated Disability Evaluation System
IET	initial entry training
MEB	Medical Evaluation Board
MTF	military treatment facility
OLS	ordinary least squares
PDRL	Permanent Disability Retirement List
PEB	Physician Evaluation Board

PEBLO	Physical Evaluation Board Liaison Officers
PPACA	Patient Protection and Affordable Care Act
PPO	preferred provider option
PTSD	post-traumatic stress disorder
QRMC	Quadrennial Review of Military Compensation
RC	Reserve Component
SCHIP	State Child Health Insurance Program
SoF-R	Status of Forces Survey of Reserve Component Personnel
SSA	Social Security Administration
TDRL	Temporary Disability Retirement List
TMA	TRICARE Management Activity
TRS	TRICARE Reserve Select
VA	Department of Veterans Affairs
VASRD	Veterans Affairs Schedule for Rating Disabilities

CHAPTER ONE

Introduction

Background

After September 11, 2001, the utilization of reserve component (RC) personnel increased dramatically and has remained high. At the beginning of 2011, more than 91,000 RC members were serving on active duty; over the decade, there have been roughly 800,000 activations. To put these numbers in context, there were only slightly more than 1 million individuals serving in RC units or as individual augmentees as of September 2010.[1]

At the same time, a decade of combat has focused the nation's attention on meeting the needs of service members—both active component (AC) and RC—whose military service has led to disability. In 2007, several study groups drew attention to inadequacies in the Disability Evaluation System (DES) and the Department of Veterans Affairs (VA) veterans disability system. Study recommendations included a major overhaul of the disability rating schedule used by the Department of Defense (DoD) and the VA, better integration of the two departments' disability evaluation processes, and a fundamental restructuring of disability compensation (Veterans' Disability Benefits Commission, 2007).

AC and RC personnel serving on active duty for more than 30 days have comprehensive healthcare coverage, but other RC members are covered only for injuries or illness sustained in the line of duty. For other conditions, they must rely on their civilian healthcare coverage—if they have such coverage. Once the necessary treatment has been provided, those whose injuries or illnesses leave them with a disability are evaluated by the DoD DES to determine whether they can continue in service or should be separated and provided with disability benefits.

Legislation passed in 1965 required the President to review military compensation every four years. In light of the critical role the reserve components have played and are likely to continue to play in the future, the President asked the 11th Quadrennial Review of Military Compensation (QRMC) to look at compensation and benefits for RC personnel. More specifically, the memo directing DoD to conduct the 11th

---

1 These figures were obtained from a 2011 DoD review of the future role of the RC.

QRMC lists four focus areas, which are important elements supporting service members who are injured or become ill:

1. Compensation for service performed in a combat zone, combat operation, or hostile fire area, or while exposed to a hostile fire event
2. Reserve and National Guard compensation and benefits in terms of how consistent they are given their current and planned utilization
3. Compensation benefits available to wounded warriors, caregivers, and survivors of fallen service members
4. Pay incentives for critical career fields, such as mental health professionals, linguists/translators, remotely-piloted-vehicle operators, and Special Operations personnel.

Objectives

As part of the 11th QRMC, RAND was asked to analyze the healthcare coverage of RC members,[2] including participation in the TRICARE Reserve Select (TRS) program, the potential effects of national health reform on coverage rates, and disability evaluation outcomes for RC members. Any consideration of healthcare coverage for RC members must take into account national health reform, specifically, the complex provisions of the Patient Protection and Affordable Care Act (PPACA). Some PPACA provisions have already taken effect—e.g., requiring coverage of young adults up to age 26 on their parents' health plans. Other provisions, including an individual insurance coverage mandate and state-run insurance exchanges, will be phased in over the next five years.

This report documents RAND's research addressing the following questions:

- What fraction of RC members have civilian healthcare coverage when they are not serving on active duty, and how do insured members differ from uninsured members? How many are getting their coverage through the TRS plan for RC members?
- What are the implications of national health reform for members' healthcare coverage? Will health reform affect TRS enrollment?
- What are the disability outcomes for wounded/injured/ill members, and are there differences in outcomes for RC and AC personnel?

[2] Dental insurance is not considered in this report. For information on dental insurance and dental readiness of RC members, see Brauner, Jackson, and Gayton, 2012.

Approach

To answer these questions, we analyzed survey data on RC members' health insurance coverage, data on enrollment in TRS, and the records of disability cases in recent years. The analysis of health reform effects draws on a microsimulation model developed to predict the effects of the individual elements of health reform on insurance status and other outcomes. These analyses are supplemented with information drawn from the relevant research literature.

Organization of This Monograph

Chapter Two discusses healthcare coverage, including current coverage, TRS enrollment, and the implications of health reform. Chapter Three describes the DES and its integration with the VA disability system and analyzes data on DES outcomes and processing time. Chapter Four presents the major findings of the study.

CHAPTER TWO

Healthcare Coverage

Introduction

All AC members have comprehensive healthcare coverage through the Military Health System while they are in service. In contrast, as part-time military personnel, RC members are guaranteed healthcare coverage only when they are activated for a period of more than 30 days and for health conditions that can be linked to their military service. At other times and for other health conditions, they must arrange for their own coverage through employer programs or other public and private options for which they may be eligible. Health insurance coverage of RC members is of public concern for two reasons: First, without insurance, members may not be able to pay for healthcare needed to maintain their medical readiness to continue in service. Second, the nation has an obligation to ensure the well-being of those who volunteer to serve in the military. Beginning in 2004, the military's health program, TRICARE, was made available to certain RC members who are willing to pay a portion of the premium. Eligibility and the terms of participation in the TRS program have gradually changed to make the program more available and attractive to members. With these changes, TRS has the potential to be an important element of the RC compensation package.

This chapter begins with background on military coverage for RC members, compares that coverage to that of AC members, and examines the relationship between medical readiness and insurance coverage. It then looks at (1) how many RC members have insurance when not activated and which members are more or less likely to be insured, (2) participation in TRS, and (3) the potential for future changes in coverage through TRS and health reform.

Eligibility for and Sources of Military Healthcare Coverage

The sources of healthcare for AC and activated RC personnel differ markedly from those for non-activated RC members. As noted above, the military services provide comprehensive healthcare for AC personnel and RC personnel serving on active duty for more than 30 days, and for their dependents. For other RC personnel, care is provided only for medical conditions sustained in the line of duty (i.e., that are caused or aggravated by the member's military service) and only for the member (not for dependents).

Healthcare for AC personnel and RC personnel activated for more than 30 days is provided through DoD's TRICARE program; all members are enrolled in the program's health maintenance organization (HMO) option, TRICARE Prime. Most healthcare for active-duty personnel is provided in military treatment facilities (MTFs); referral to a civilian provider is arranged when appropriate MTF care is not available. The cost of care, regardless of where it is provided, is fully covered by TRICARE.

Full TRICARE coverage for the activated RC members and their dependents begins when their orders are issued or up to 180 days before activation and remains in effect for 180 days after deactivation. Continuing care after the 180-day post-activation period is available only for health conditions that are determined to be line-of-duty, consistent with the policies for non-activated RC members. Members must arrange follow-up care for conditions not in the line of duty through their civilian health plans, if any.

Non-activated RC members with line-of-duty conditions are usually cared for through TRICARE's civilian provider network. This network is extensive in geographic areas that have sizable TRICARE beneficiary populations (including active-duty dependents and retired military and their dependents); it is less extensive in some other geographic areas, although many VA health facilities also belong to the TRICARE network.

Finally, RC members who return from deployment to the Iraq and Afghanistan theaters are immediately eligible for care in VA facilities for up to five years.[1] They must enroll in the VA system, but enrollment is now done automatically as part of the demobilization process. Once enrolled, they are eligible for a full range of healthcare services in the VA's 152 medical centers and 798 outpatient clinics.[2]

Line of Duty

As described in Chapter Three, the line-of-duty rule governs AC members' eligibility for disability separation or retirement (and associated benefits); however, it is rarely a factor in eligibility for healthcare, because most AC members enter with a clean bill of health and are always on duty while they are in service. Thus, the line-of-duty requirement for healthcare eligibility applies primarily to health conditions RC members develop when they are not activated or are activated for 30 days or less.

---

[1] The period of eligibility was extended from two years to five years in 2008. Eligibility continues after the five-year eligibility period ends, although the VA does reevaluate individuals' enrollment status according to enrollment policy and priority.

[2] The focus of this discussion is *member* health insurance coverage. A member's dependents are also covered by TRICARE when he or she is activated, and TRS enrollees may elect to cover their dependents as well as themselves. Otherwise, dependents are not covered by either TRICARE or the VA.

Determining whether an RC member's health condition was incurred (or aggravated) in the line of duty is relatively straightforward when he or she is injured during a period of active military service or while in training or participating in inactive-duty training or active-duty training. Similarly, injuries incurred at other times may be readily ruled out unless they are linked to a service-related condition. Some non-injuries may also be easily linked to service—e.g., post-traumatic stress disorder (PTSD) among members who have been deployed to a combat theater or conditions resulting from known exposures or infectious diseases endemic in a location where the member served. However, many medical conditions, including common chronic conditions such as diabetes, are not considered service-connected unless there is evidence that the condition was aggravated by service. Others, such as chronic musculoskeletal conditions that develop over time (bad backs and knees), may be difficult to attribute to military service. How many RC members can get a line-of-duty decision that makes them eligible for care through TRICARE and how many must rely instead on their other insurance or self-financing is unknown, but RC members clearly need their own health insurance to ensure healthcare coverage.

TRS Eligibility and Enrollee Cost

In 2004, premium-based TRICARE coverage was temporarily extended to non-activated reservists who were unemployed or ineligible for employer-sponsored insurance, and TRS was established as a permanent benefit the following year. As Table 2.1 shows, eligibility requirements and the premium contribution required for enrollment varied during the program's initial years. Since 2007, all Selected Reserve members who are not eligible for Federal Employee Health Benefits (FEHB) through their civilian employment may enroll in TRS for individual or family coverage. TRS is based on the preferred provider option (PPO) in TRICARE (TRICARE Standard/Extra) and requires a premium contribution equal to 28 percent of the estimated total plan cost. Initially, premium levels for individual and family coverage were based on the costs of the nationwide Blue Cross/Blue Shield Plan in FEHB. The premiums decreased in 2009 (as shown in Table 2.1), when experience showed that actual TRS costs were considerably lower than costs in the FEHB plan and in response to low rates of enrollment (Government Accountability Office, 2007; TRICARE Management Activity, 2011).

TRS enrollees are eligible for care in the MTFs when space is available for them or for care from civilian healthcare providers. MTF care may not be practical for enrollees who live too far from an MTF. Even for those who live in an MTF service area, the MTF may not have availability to treat them. The MTFs allocate their treatment capacity according to prescribed beneficiary-group priorities. DoD policy establishes a hierarchy of five priority groups for MTF care; TRS enrollees are in the fourth category, below AC members, RC members serving on active duty or seeking care for a line-of-duty problem, and all other beneficiaries who have enrolled in TRICARE

Table 2.1
TRS Eligibility and Premium Contributions, 2005–2011

Year	Eligibility	Annual Premium
2005	Members of the Selected Reserve who • Served on active duty in support of a contingency operation on or after 9/11 for ≥ 90 days • Agree to serve in the Selected Reserves for the entire period of TRS coverage chosen (up to 1 year of coverage for each 90 days of active service) • Use the one-time enrollment opportunity at the end of active service unless called to active duty again	$900 for individuals, $2,796 for families
2006	Restructured with tiered premium subsidies: • Tier 1: Same as in 2005 but enrollment period is expanded to 90 days post–active duty • Tier 2: Unemployed or ineligible for employer insurance • Tier 3: All other Selected Reservists not eligible for FEHB	*Tier 1: 28%* $972 for individuals, $3,036 for families *Tier 2: 50%* $1,743 for individuals, $5,417 for families *Tier 3: 85%* $2,964 for individuals, $9,209 for families
2007–2008	All Selected Reserve members who are not eligible for FEHB	$972 for individuals, $3,063 for families
2009	All Selected Reserve members who are not eligible for FEHB	$570 for individuals, $2,162 for families
2010–2011	All Selected Reserve members who are not eligible for FEHB	$638 for individuals, $2,373 for families

Prime (the HMO option). Given their relatively low priority, TRS enrollees rarely have MTF care available to them; thus, their usual source of care is civilian providers. The out-of-pocket costs for civilian care in TRS are the same as those for active-duty dependents electing the same PPO option (Standard/Extra):

- $50/$100 annual deductible for individuals/families for junior enlisted personnel (E-4 and below); $150/$300 for all others
- 15/20 percent cost-sharing for in-network/out-of-network providers, respectively
- $1,000 catastrophic limit on out-of-pocket costs (excluding premium contribution) per family.

Relationship Between Health Insurance Coverage and Health

As mentioned earlier, one motive for offering health insurance to RC members may be the expectation that insurance will enhance the members' medical readiness to perform their military duties. A key medical readiness requirement is having no deployment-limiting medical condition; a second requirement, completing an annual self-report health status form, is designed to identify any such problem for evaluation and treatment. Members with health insurance may be more likely to be medically ready if they get regular preventive care leading to early identification and effective treatment of health problems or if they seek care earlier when symptoms of a health problem arise. However, in a largely healthy population such as the RC, health insurance may have little effect on health status.

The effect of health insurance on the medical readiness of RC members has not been studied (Hosek, 2010). However, there are hundreds of observational studies that examine insurance status and health outcomes, most of which do not address the causal effect of insurance on health. Three decades ago, a random, controlled trial—the RAND Health Insurance Experiment—measured the effects of different levels of cost-sharing on healthcare utilization and health outcomes in a representative population under the age of 65. The main health finding was the following:

> For persons with poor vision and for low-income persons with high blood pressure, free care brought an improvement (vision better by 0.2 Snellen lines, diastolic blood pressure lower by 3 mm Hg); better control of blood pressure reduced the calculated risk of early death among those at high risk. For the average participant, as well as for subgroups differing in income and initial health status, no significant effects were detected on eight other measures of health status and health habits. (Brook et al., 1983)

Two articles that review more recent evidence for a causal effect of health insurance on health outcomes (Freeman et al., 2008; Levy and Meltzer, 2008) also find some evidence of positive health effects of insurance in vulnerable populations. Levy and Meltzer focused on studies of natural experiments (e.g., arising from major policy shifts such as the enactment of Medicare and expansions of Medicaid). They report:

> The evidence available to date conclusively demonstrates that health insurance improves the health of vulnerable subpopulations such as infants, children, and individuals with AIDS and that it can improve specific measures of health such as control of high blood pressure for a broader population of adults, especially those with low income. For most of the population at risk of being uninsured (adults ages 19 to 50), we have limited reliable evidence on how health insurance affects health. This lack of evidence and the resulting lack of consensus indicate that to summarize the effects of health insurance on health is, inevitably, to misrepresent.

Freeman et al. cite two studies with more objective measures of health outcomes that show health insurance causes an improvement in self-reported health status in a general population of adults; the studies consider subpopulations with specific health problems, and they similarly find positive health effects of insurance.

The Institute of Medicine has published a series of reports on health insurance in the United States. The most recent report updates its earlier assessments of the decline in the number of Americans with health insurance and the effects of not having insurance on healthcare utilization and health outcomes (Institute of Medicine, 2009). That report concludes that children benefit substantially from health insurance, adults with health insurance are more likely to get effective preventive care and be diagnosed with later-stage cancers, and individuals with chronic illness and no health insurance have worse outcomes.

These reviews provide considerable evidence that health insurance leads to better health outcomes for children and adults at risk for poor health. Insured adults are more likely to seek care and discover that they have developed (chronic) health conditions. However, most of the evidence linking health insurance to health outcomes comes from subpopulations that are not similar to most RC members, especially to uninsured RC members (see below). Therefore, the current evidence does not support a conclusion about the likely effects of health insurance on the medical readiness of RC members.

A study currently under way may add new information about the effects of health insurance in a non-aged adult population. Taking advantage of a lottery employed in a recent expansion of the Oregon Medicaid program, a research team is conducting the equivalent of a controlled trial on the effects of insuring previously uninsured, non-aged adults with incomes just above the federal poverty level. Initial results indicate that newly insured adults substantially increase their healthcare use and report less financial strain and improved health and well-being (Finkelstein et al., 2011). Future results will provide objective measures of the effects of Medicaid coverage on health.

The research literature does not yet address the relationship between health insurance and medical readiness of RC members. However, the literature does suggest that their children are likely to be in better health if they have insurance.

Rate of Health Insurance Coverage Among RC Members

Status of Forces Survey

The Status of Forces Survey of Reserve Component Personnel (SoF-R) periodically includes a question about RC members' health insurance coverage. The survey is administered to a sample of Selected Reserve members twice a year; every two years, the survey asks respondents whether they have health/medical insurance.[3] Respondents who are activated at the time of the survey are asked whether they had health insurance before they were called to active duty. The most recent survey that includes information on health insurance coverage was fielded in January 2011 by the Defense Manpower Data Center (DMDC).[4] A stratified random sample for the module containing the health insurance question included 120,724 members who had at least six months of service and were below the rank of flag officer. Of the sample, 90.8 percent were located, and the completion rate of the located respondents was 20.5 percent. One-third of the original sample received a survey module that included questions on

---

[3] The question does not specify the sources of insurance the respondent should consider when answering. TRS enrollees do report having insurance on this question.

[4] The survey fielded in January 2011 is not publicly available. RAND was provided with an early release of the database and an interim codebook for this study.

health insurance coverage. We deleted the respondents who were not given this module and two groups of respondents who serve full time for an extended period in the military as military or civilian personnel: Active Guard Reserve (AGR) members, who are covered by TRICARE, and Military Technicians, who are covered by the FEHB program. Our final working sample comprised 7,825 respondents who had responses for health insurance coverage and the other variables used in our analyses. Weights provided with the data adjust for differences across subgroups in the sampling rate and nonresponse rate.[5]

The survey results show that 70 percent of Selected Reserve members, excluding AGRs and military technicians, had health insurance in 2011. Figure 2.1 plots the percentage that reported having insurance, by military service, for junior enlisted personnel (E-1–E-4), senior enlisted personnel (E-5–E-9), and all warrant and commissioned officers. There is some variation across the services, especially for junior enlisted personnel, and the rates of insurance coverage are higher for senior enlisted personnel and officers in all the services.

Health insurance coverage rates in the RC population mirror the rates in the general population. We compared the 2008 SoF-R data with data for the general adult population from the Current Population Survey (CPS) for the same year. In the CPS,

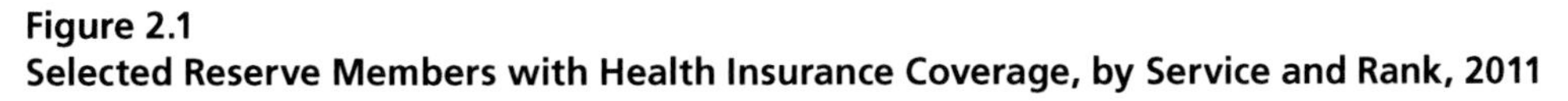

Figure 2.1
Selected Reserve Members with Health Insurance Coverage, by Service and Rank, 2011

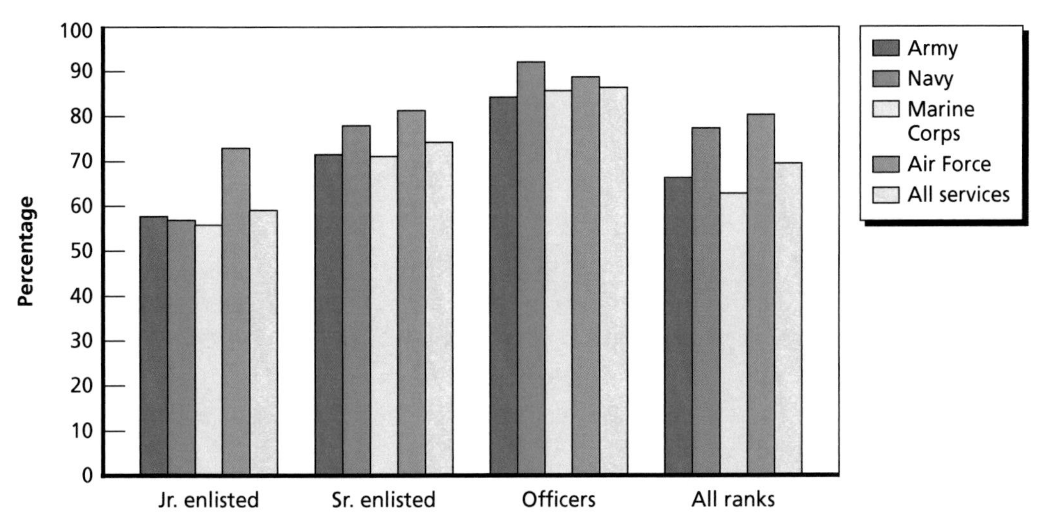

SOURCE: SoF-R, 2011 (weighted).
RAND *MG1157-2.1*

[5] Detailed documentation of this survey is provided in Defense Manpower Data Center, 2009. The weights adjust for observed differences in response rate (e.g., by rank, gender) but not for unobserved differences. If nonrespondents would not have answered the questions the same way respondents with the same observed characteristics did, the weights do not eliminate nonresponse bias in the results.

the insured rate varied from 71 percent for adults 18 to 24 years of age to 84 percent for those 45 to 54 years of age (U.S. Census Bureau, undated). To compare health insurance coverage in the RC population with that of a roughly comparable U.S. population, we multiplied the percentage with health insurance by age group in the CPS by the percentage of Selected Reserve members in the same age group. In the reweighted CPS data, 76 percent were insured—the same fraction that reported having insurance in the SoF-R for the same year.[6]

Considerable public attention has focused on declining rates of health insurance in the United States. The CPS data (matched to the age distribution in the Selected Reserve) show a decrease in the insured rate from 80 percent in 2000 to 76 in 2008. In contrast, the insured rate among members of the Selected Reserve remained constant over the same time period—in the 2000 Survey of Reserve Component Personnel, 74 percent of respondents reported that they had insurance (Hosek, 2010)—the same as in 2008.[7] More recent CPS data show a further erosion of insurance coverage in the civilian population between 2008 and 2009 as economic conditions worsened during the recent recession. Similarly, the SoF-R shows a decline in coverage rates over the two years between survey waves (from 74 percent to 70 percent).

Factors Associated with Having Health Insurance Coverage

We used multivariate regression to determine the association between member characteristics and health insurance coverage. The dependent variable indicated whether each respondent to the SoF-R survey reported having health insurance, and the explanatory variables were service component, rank, gender, race/ethnicity, education, marital status, whether the respondent had children ages 0–13 or 14–22, employment, type and size of firm if employed, and whether the respondent was a student. Variable means and regression coefficients and standard errors, which were estimated in a linear probability model, are shown in Tables A.1 and A.2 in the Appendix.

Figure 2.2 shows selected results from the regression analysis. Each set of bars in the figure represents the difference between the indicated group and the comparison group. For example, the top bar indicates that personnel in the top three enlisted ranks are four percentage points *more likely* than officers to have health insurance.[8] However, lower-ranking enlisted personnel are less likely to have health insurance. The survey file used for this analysis did not include age or income, so these results for rank reflect the

6 A more detailed comparison controlling for age, gender, marital status, number of children, and income also showed that the rates for reservists are the same as those for the comparable general population (see the analysis of the effects of health reform below).

7 A change in the health insurance questions may have affected responses over time. The 2000 survey included several questions about specific sources of health insurance that may have led to more complete reporting of coverage.

8 Standard errors for all regression coefficients are included in the Appendix tables. This coefficient just misses being statistically significant at the 0.05 level.

Figure 2.2
Differences Between Categories of RC Members Who Have Health Insurance

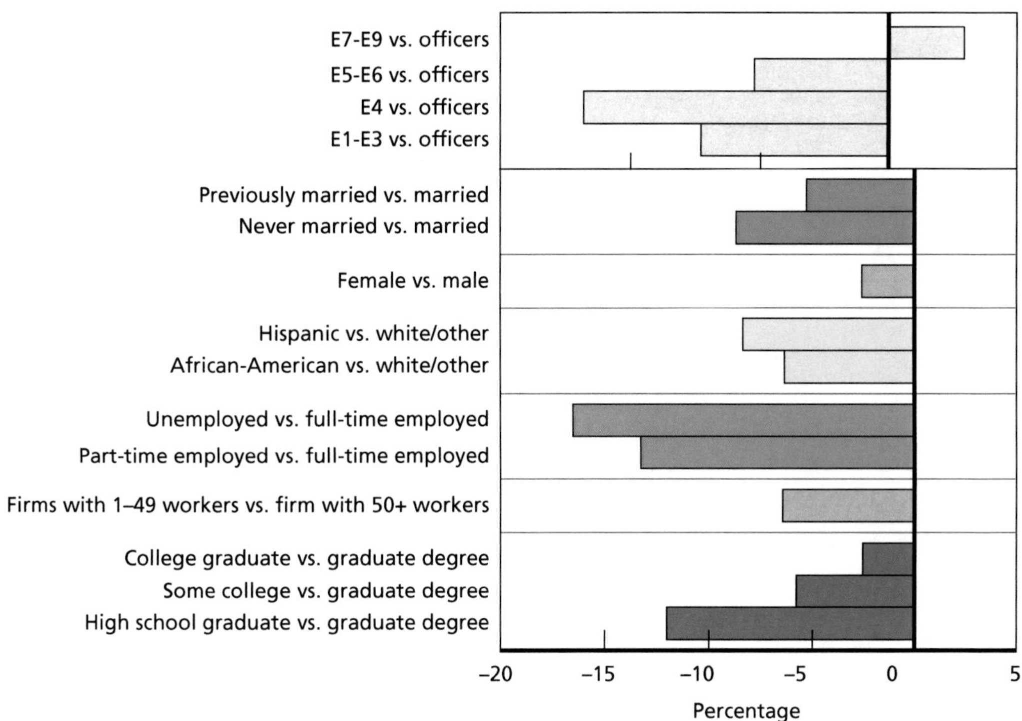

SOURCE: SoF-R, 2008.
RAND *MG1157-2.2*

strong relationship typically seen between the characteristics of these rank groups and insurance coverage—namely, that young adults and lower-income individuals (unless they are eligible for Medicaid) are less likely to be insured. In earlier years of the SoF-R, the most junior enlisted personnel (E-1–E-3) had the lowest coverage rate, but in 2011 their coverage rate was somewhat higher than that for personnel in the next higher rank (E-4). They were also the only rank group that did not experience a decline in health insurance coverage rate between the 2008 and 2011 surveys. A provision of the federal health reform legislation implemented in September 2010 mandated that health plans offering dependent coverage extend eligibility to age 26. Previously, eligibility varied by state but typically did not include young adults unless they were financially dependent or attending college. It seems likely that more of the lowest-ranking RC members are now insured because they have been able to continue their parents' coverage.

In employer-based health insurance systems, employment status is strongly associated with being insured, as one might expect. Benefits are often unavailable to part-time workers, and among RC members, the difference between full-time and part-time workers in the proportion with health insurance was 18 percentage points. Members who were unemployed at the time of the survey were also less likely to have insurance, but the gap was smaller than it was for part-time workers. Those working for very small employers were also less likely to have insurance. Small employers are much less likely to offer their employees health insurance than large employers are. In 2010, only 55 percent of firms employing fewer than ten workers offered health benefits of any kind, whereas 76 percent of firms with ten to 24 workers and 90 percent of larger firms offered benefits (Kaiser Family Foundation and Health Research and Educational Trust, 2010). Finally, controlling for employment status and employer size, there was no difference associated with the type of employer (i.e., public, nonprofit, private, own or family business).

Personal and family characteristics also were associated with members' probability of having health insurance. As shown in Figure 2.2, previously married and single members were less likely to have insurance than married members. Men were less likely than women to have health insurance, as were those who had less education. Controlling for all these other variables, whether the member had children was not associated with having insurance; in simple tabulations, however, those with children are more likely to be insured. Like military rank, these personal characteristics are related to characteristics not included in the SoF-R data, especially income. Other studies have shown a strong relationship between income and being insured (Gruber, 2008; Abraham and Feldman, 2010). The SoF-R also lacks information on health status, another important factor in health insurance decisions.

To summarize these results, the SoF-R data show that RC members without health insurance in late 2008 tended to be in the junior enlisted ranks, less well-educated, single, likely to have lower incomes, and likely to be working part time or for a small employer. Many of them lacked insurance either because they were not offered employer-based health insurance or because they chose not to participate in their employer's plan. The most likely reason for nonparticipation is the size of the premium contribution, which has been increasing. Across firms of all sizes in 2010, the average annual premium was $900 for single coverage and $5,000 for family coverage (Kaiser Family Foundation and Health Research and Educational Trust, 2010).

Enrollment in TRS

To examine TRS enrollment, we used data from the Defense Enrollment Eligibility Reporting System (DEERS), the official enrollment file for TRICARE. DEERS has less information about members than the SoF-R survey has, but it is more current and its enrollment data are more reliable. We use DEERS enrollment information, along with member and dependent characteristics, for June 2008 and June 2010. This was 6 months before and 18 months after a 30- to 40-percent decrease in premium contribution, which probably accelerated the increase in enrollment in what is still a new program. Using consistently scrambled individual identifiers, the DEERS file was linked to a DoD civilian personnel data file for the same months to identify RC members who, as DoD civilian employees, are eligible for the FEHB and not for TRS. We excluded these individuals from the eligible population in calculating enrollment rates.

TRS enrollment increased by 239 percent in the two years between 2008 and 2010 to over 60,000 Selected Reserve members (Figure 2.3). There was almost no voluntary disenrollment between the two years; most of the 2008 enrollees who left TRS were either activated and had their enrollment switched to TRICARE or left the Selected Reserve and became ineligible. Most of the added enrollees in 2010 were already serving members, but a sizable number were new RC entrants. Six percent of members who entered between June 2008 and June 2010 enrolled in TRS, and 8 percent of members who were already serving in 2008 had enrolled by 2010. TRS enrollment continues to increase; by December 31, 2010, it had risen to 67,259 members.[9]

Enrollment rates are highest for commissioned officers and among those who are married and have children under the age of 14 (Table 2.2). This is not the population of RC members likely to be uninsured in the SoF-R survey data.[10]

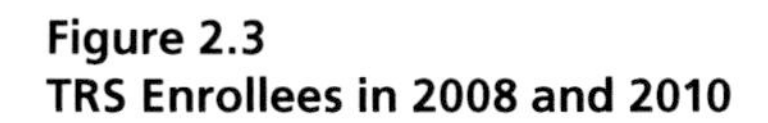

Figure 2.3
TRS Enrollees in 2008 and 2010

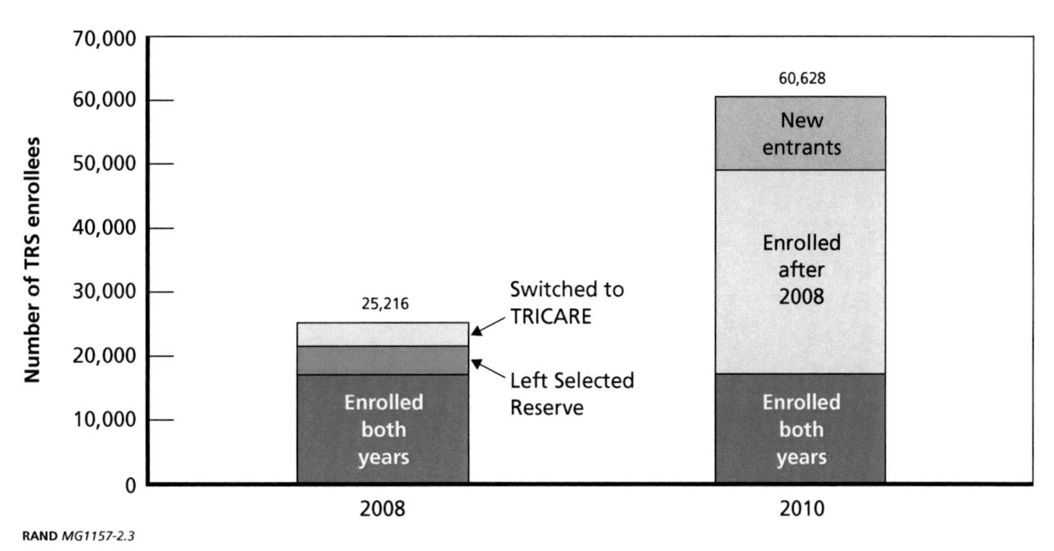

RAND *MG1157-2.3*

---

[9] Jody W. Donohoo, "Total Force + TRICARE® = MHS Commitment to . . . Reserve Warriors and Their Families: Before, During and After Activation," unpublished survey results presented at the 2011 Military Health System Conference.

[10] More direct evidence of the value of TRS for uninsured RC members comes from the 2000 SoF-R, which asked about willingness to pay for DoD-sponsored health insurance if it were offered. At that time, only 10 percent of the respondents who were uninsured valued an insurance option at more than $100 per month ($131 in 2011 dollars). This is more than the TRS premium for single coverage but considerably less than the premium for family coverage.

Table 2.2
TRS Enrollment Rate, by Member Characteristics, June 2010

Characteristic	Percent Enrolled
Rank	
E-1–E-4	4
E-5–E-9	10
Warrant officer	10
Commissioned officer	13
Gender	
Female	4
Male	8
Marital status	
Single	1
Married	14
Child age 0–13	
No	3
Yes	16

Among respondents to a spring 2008 survey of Selected Reserve members conducted by the TRICARE Management Activity (TMA), the most common reason for enrolling in TRS, cited by 69 percent of enrollees, was that it was "more affordable."[11] Only 31 percent indicated that they had "no other healthcare alternatives." Approximately half of the enrollees who responded to this survey reported that they had another health insurance option, compared with 70 percent of the respondents not enrolled in TRS. These results indicate that TRS was more attractive to members who lack other options, but that a substantial fraction of enrollees are opting for TRS instead of employer-provided coverage.[12]

The cost of public health insurance is higher when there is a crowd-out of private health insurance, which occurs when individuals pass up or drop private health insurance they are eligible for and enroll in the public program instead. Crowd-out has been studied primarily for Medicaid, and the studies have produced differing results; data from an expansion of the State Child Health Insurance Program (SCHIP) to higher income levels (Gruber and Simon, 2008) show a substantial rate of crowd-out, approximately 60 percent. There is also evidence of crowd-out in military retirees under the age

[11] Unpublished survey results presented at the 2011 Military Health System Conference.

[12] The response rate for this survey was only 18 percent, and these appear to be unweighted results. The SoF-R results, collected six months later, indicate that three-quarters of all Selected Reserve members have health insurance—a higher fraction than reported having any civilian option in the TMA survey. Health insurance questions can be difficult for respondents to answer accurately, and these two surveys word the health insurance questions differently.

of 65, the other military population likely to have a civilian health insurance option. A 2006 survey of civilian health insurance eligibility and coverage of non-elderly retirees, all of whom are enrolled in TRICARE, showed that almost four-fifths are eligible for civilian insurance, but only half of them actually enroll in a civilian plan (Mariano et al., 2007); most of those not selecting civilian insurance enroll in TRICARE's Prime option, which requires a small annual premium but has only minimal cost-sharing.

Overall, although TRS may be enrolling some Selected Reserve members who would otherwise be uninsured, the rapidly growing number of enrollees appears to include a significant fraction who take up TRS instead of employer insurance because TRS is more affordable. Recall that the premium contribution for TRS is roughly half the average contribution for employer plans. Enrollment in TRS can be expected to increase further as eligible RC members learn about it.

DoD's annual cost per RC member enrolling in TRS is almost $2,300 for single coverage and almost $8,500 for family coverage. To put this cost in context, an enlisted member joining the reserves after an initial term of active service (e.g., rank E-4, four years of service) is paid about $4,600 for one drill day per month and 14 days of summer training. If significant numbers were to enroll in TRS, this would represent a large increase in the cost of compensation. For RC members, the added benefit would equal the difference between the premiums and out-of-pocket costs for care in TRS and those of their other sources of health insurance (for those willing to pay the premium cost). It is not clear whether TRS will have a significant impact on recruiting and retention. However, research has generally shown some relationship between health insurance and job decisions in the civilian labor market.[13]

Potential Effects of Health Reform on Health Insurance Coverage for RC Members

PPACA contains several provisions that expand the health insurance options relevant to RC members (The Commonwealth Fund, 2011). The first of these provisions allows young adults up to age 26 to be covered under their parents' insurance, effective immediately. The others will be effective in 2014:

- Medicaid eligibility for all individuals at up to 133 percent of the federal poverty level (FPL)
- Health insurance exchanges offering a choice of standardized plans to small businesses and individuals without employer coverage

---

[13] For example, recent studies have shown that fathers whose children became eligible for SCHIP were more likely to change jobs (Bansak and Raphael, 2008) and that job turnover is higher in industries with higher rates of employer health insurance (Ellis and Ma, 2011). Earlier, Gruber and Madrian (2002) reviewed the literature and concluded that availability of health insurance does affect job decisions.

- Sliding-scale subsidies for insurance purchased through the exchanges for families with incomes of up to 400 percent of the FPL
- Mandated coverage for individuals and businesses with at least 50 employees, with penalties for noncompliance.

The subsidies will be set at a level that caps the cost of health plans offered in the exchanges to a percentage of income that increases with the level of income relative to the FPL (Table 2.3).

The individual penalty for failure to insure will be phased in over three years; in 2016, it will be equal to $695 or 2.5 percent of applicable income, up to a maximum of three times that amount per family, or $2,085. There are exemptions from the penalty for individuals who (1) cannot find coverage at a cost to them of less than 8 percent of income, (2) have incomes below the threshold for paying income taxes (currently $9,350 for single coverage and $18,700 for a couple), or have been uncovered for less than three months. The individual mandate is being challenged in the courts, with differing decisions at the lower court levels that will require a Supreme Court decision about whether the provision is constitutional. The employer penalty is expected to have little impact because almost all employers with 50 workers or more already offer insurance; however, some employers may be forced to improve the coverage they now offer.

Figure 2.4 plots the maximum cost for TRS and the maximum annual cost of health insurance that will be purchased through the state exchanges when they are implemented in 2014 for those eligible for subsidies. The premium calculations are based on the 2011 FPL to make them comparable with the current TRS premiums. TRS costs are lower than the subsidized costs in the health exchanges at all income levels above 150 percent of the FPL ($16,000 for a single person and $34,000 for a family of four in 2011). For single coverage, the current TRS premium is $100 lower

Table 2.3
Premium and Out-of-Pocket Limits in State Health Insurance Exchanges Under PPACA

	Maximum Share of Income for	
Percentage of FPL	**Premium Contribution (%)**	**Annual Out-of-Pocket Cost**
Up to 133	2.0	
133–150	3.0–4.0	$1,983 for individuals, $3,967 for families
150–200	4.0–6.3	
200–250	6.3–8.05	$2,975 for individuals, $5,950 for families
250–300	8.05–9.5	
300–400	9.5	$3,967 for individuals, $7,933 for families
Above 400	No limit specified	$5,950 for individuals, $11,900 for families

Figure 2.4
Comparison of Maximum Cost per Year of Health Exchange Plans and TRS

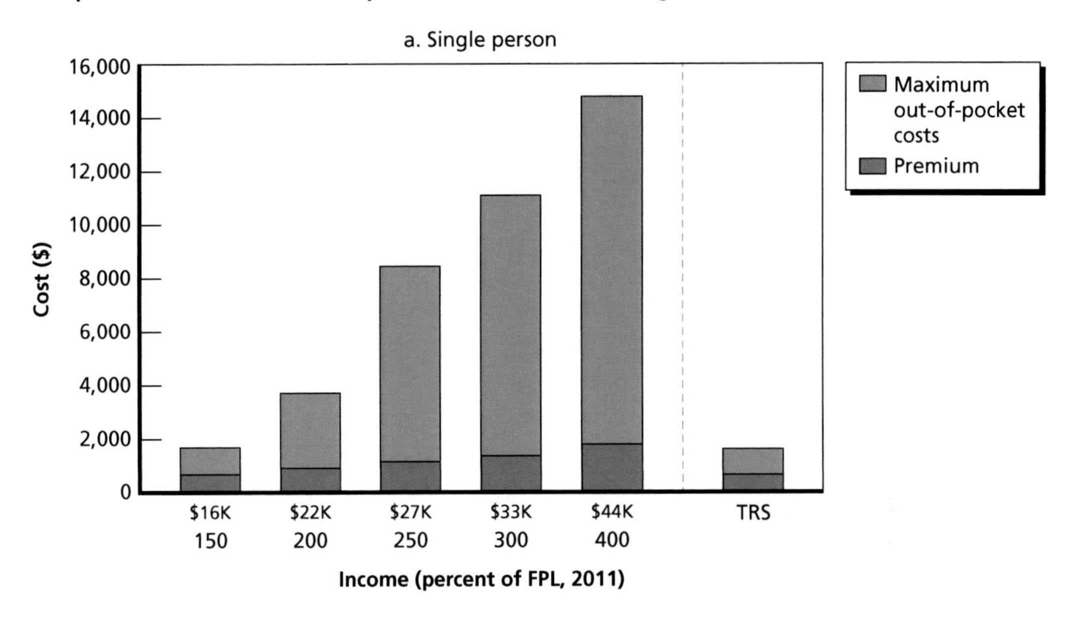

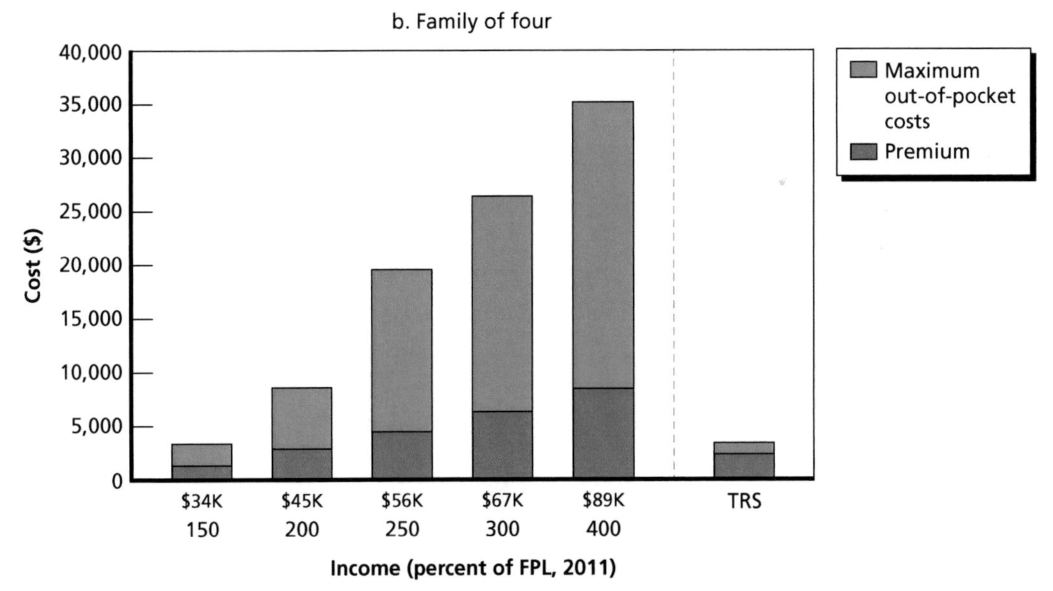

RAND *MG1157-2.4*

than the penalty for not having coverage under health reform, and for family coverage, it is approximately $300 higher. It seems reasonable to expect that if this provision is ultimately implemented, many currently uninsured RC members will turn to TRS instead of paying the penalty. A similar mandate and penalty in Massachusetts was effective in inducing previously uninsured and healthy individuals to purchase insurance (Chandra et al., 2011).

To examine the potential effects of health reform on health insurance coverage of RC members, we used the RAND COMPARE microsimulation model of health reform (Girosi et al., 2009). The model projects how individuals, households, and firms are likely to respond to healthcare policy changes, including the ones included in PPACA, based on the economic theory of health decisionmaking and accumulated evidence from more modest policy changes (e.g., changes in Medicaid eligibility).

The COMPARE model's simulation of the effects of PPACA was used to predict the change in the rate of health insurance coverage for RC members. The calculation was based on a decomposition of the RC population into subgroups defined by age (under 25, 25–34, 35–44, 45 and over), gender, marital status (single or married), number of children (0, 1, 2, 3, 4, 5, 6+), and rank (enlisted or officer). After combining subgroups with fewer than 100 members, we had 137 subgroups. For each subgroup, we obtained information on combined member and spouse earnings from a dataset created at the Social Security Administration (SSA) by merging DoD personnel records with Medicare earnings data. For each subgroup of RC members, SSA provided the percentage whose annual family (member plus spouse) earnings were in each of ten earnings groups defined relative to the FPL: up to 1.33 times the FPL, 1.34 to 1.50, 1.51 to 2.00, 2.01 to 2.50, 2.51 to 3.00, 3.01 to 3.50, 3.51 to 4.00, 4.01 to 5.00, 5.01 to 6.00, and over 6.00. Using this information, the 137 subgroups were subdivided by income level. The COMPARE model yielded predictions of the change in the percentage of RC members with health insurance after health reform in each subgroup. In most cases, the insurance coverage of dependents is the same as that for RC members. Here, we report only the predicted coverage rates for members.

First, we generated an estimate of the current (pre-reform) health insurance coverage rate for RC members. This provided a test of the applicability of the microsimulation model to the RC population and a baseline estimate to compare with the post-reform estimate. For the overall population, the microsimulation model estimated an insured rate of 76 percent—the same rate that was estimated from the 2008 SoF-R. The model's post-reform insured prediction is substantially higher, at 89 percent. This prediction does not factor in the availability of TRS; it considers only the standard insurance options after reform is implemented.

Figure 2.5 shows the predicted post-reform sources of health insurance for RC member households. Employers will remain the primary source of health insurance, but some employers will arrange for employee coverage through the health insurance exchanges instead of traditional sources.[14] Individual purchases through the exchanges and expanded Medicaid eligibility account for most of the remaining coverage. Of

[14] The fraction of households obtaining health insurance through employers is predicted to increase slightly, consistent with most analyses of the effects of health reform.

Figure 2.5
Predicted Source of Post-Health-Reform Health Insurance for RC Member Households

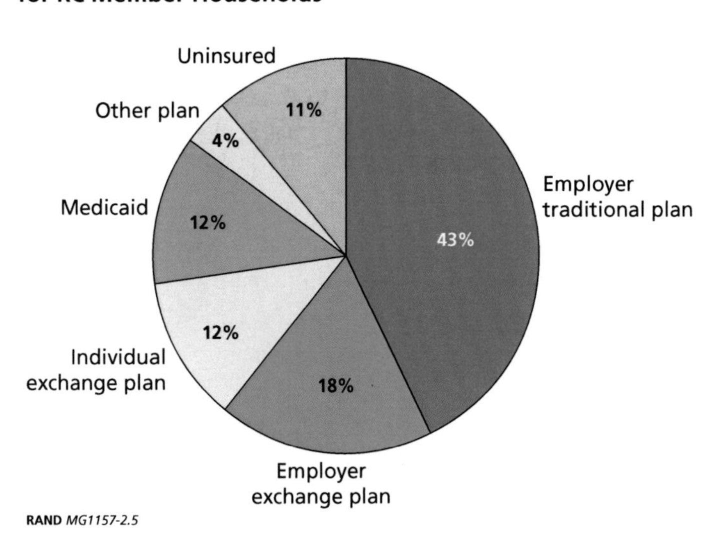

those predicted to purchase individual coverage through the exchanges (12 percent of RC households), four-fifths would qualify for a subsidy based on SSA family earnings data. Nevertheless, almost all of these households would be better off taking up TRS instead. As is true today, many predicted to be in employer plans may also find TRS more attractive. Some who would newly qualify for Medicaid may prefer to pay the premium for TRS. Finally, as discussed above, those who pay income taxes will face a penalty for not having insurance. RC members would be better off enrolling in TRS than paying the penalty.[15]

Summary

When activated for more than 30 days, RC members have the same comprehensive healthcare coverage that AC members have through TRICARE. TRICARE eligibility begins when the order to activate is processed and ends 180 days after deactivation. For RC members who are not activated for more than 30 days, the military provides care only for health problems that are incurred or aggravated in the line of duty. RC members must rely on civilian health insurance for other health problems. The 2011 SoF-R reveals that 30 percent of Selected Reserve members lack health insurance. The rate for RC members is the same as that for a comparable civilian population.

[15] Those eligible to enroll in the VA health system may be able to avoid paying a penalty for their own lack of health insurance, but they would still face a penalty if they have uncovered family members.

The TRS program was initiated to offer insurance for RC members who lack a civilian option, and both TRS eligibility and affordability have changed significantly in recent years. TRS enrollment grew rapidly after the changes were implemented and was 8 percent of the eligible population in June 2010. While it is possible that insurance coverage has not declined in this population because of the availability of TRS, the evidence suggests that quite a few enrollees have access to civilian insurance that they find less attractive. Further, the characteristics of TRS enrollees do not match well with the characteristics of uninsured RC members.

Although at present TRS may not be significantly reducing the number of uninsured members, this may change if an individual insurance mandate and associated penalties are implemented in 2014–2016 in accordance with PPACA. By itself, health reform would substantially increase the coverage rate in the RC population. However, financially, TRS compares favorably with the health insurance plans that will be offered by the state health exchanges, even for those at lower income levels who are eligible for subsidies in the exchanges. TRS premiums for single and family coverage are, at worst, only slightly higher than the penalty for not having insurance under health reform. There is a good chance that once health reform is implemented, TRS enrollment will increase substantially. This could make it very difficult to achieve the goal of controlling DoD's health costs.

CHAPTER THREE

Disability Outcomes for Reserve Component Members

Introduction

Military personnel—both AC and RC—who develop a medical condition that may interfere with their ability to meet medical standards for continued service are referred to their service Disability Evaluation System (DES) for further evaluation, and if they are found to be no longer medically fit, for disability evaluation leading to possible compensation. Personnel who have a disability because of their military service are also eligible for disability benefits from the VA after they leave service.

This chapter begins with an overview of the multistage military DES, including evaluation of medical fitness to serve, disability evaluation and rating, and disability benefits awarded based on DES outcomes. This overview concludes with a brief description of the VA's disability system and recent efforts to coordinate the evaluation processes of DoD and the VA. Finally, we present an analysis of the dispositions and processing times for DES cases initiated in fiscal years 2007–2010.

Overview of the Military Disability Evaluation System

The secretary of each branch of the military is responsible for conducting disability evaluations of that service's personnel.[1] As Figure 3.1 illustrates, the process involves a number of steps, including, in some cases, a line-of-duty investigation, a Medical Evaluation Board (MEB), and a Physician Evaluation Board (PEB). For active-duty personnel (including RC members serving on active duty), the disability evaluation process generally begins at the MTF providing care for the medical condition. Once the medical provider determines that a service member has received the maximum benefit from

[1] Policies and procedures for the Physical Disability System are provided in DoD Instruction 1332.38, dated November 14, 1996, and incorporating Change 1, July 10, 2006. A later revision is contained in a memorandum, Directive-Type Memorandum (DIM) on Implementing Disability-Related Provisions of the National Defense Authorization Act of 2008 (Pub L. I 10-181), from the Under Secretary of Defense for Personnel and Readiness, dated March 13, 2008.

Figure 3.1
Military DES

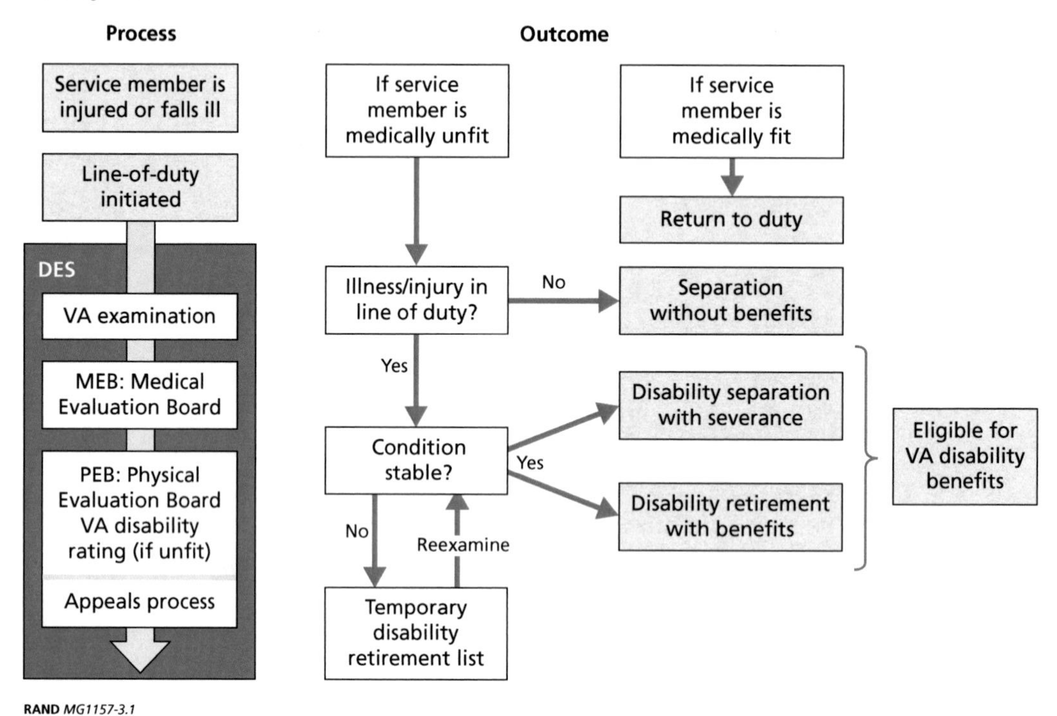

RAND *MG1157-3.1*

medical care for his or her injuries, it refers the member to the DES. Members referred to the DES have one of four basic outcomes. They are either

- Medically fit and returned to duty
- Medically separated from the military but not eligible for disability benefits
- Separated with a lower disability rating qualifying for disability severance pay
- Retired with a higher disability rating qualifying for lifetime disability benefits.

Line-of-Duty Investigation

A formal line-of-duty investigation may be required prior to referral to the DES to determine whether the condition was incurred or aggravated by military service and qualifies for military disability benefits. A formal investigation is required if the medical condition may have

- Developed in "doubtful" circumstances or may be the result of misconduct or negligence, including alcohol or drug abuse or conduct leading to charges under the Uniform Code of Military Justice
- Occurred while the member was absent from duty
- Existed prior to service.

As discussed in Chapter Two, the requirement for a determination that the medical condition was sustained in the line of duty constitutes an important difference in applying the DES for RC members. Line of duty is presumed for both AC and RC personnel and is rebutted if an investigation concludes that one of the three circumstances above applies. Since AD members are continuously in service from the time they are found fit at accession, it is unlikely that their medical conditions are preexisting and not aggravated during their service. Among RC members, intermitent service means that their medical conditions are more likely to be preexisting.[2] In 2008, the policy was altered to require "compelling" evidence to set aside the presumption for conditions identified after 30 days of active service for members with more than six months' active service. The same presumption does not exist for RC members identified as having a medical condition when not on extended active service.

Procedures for determining line of duty are established by each military service. Except when an investigation is required, the unit commander makes the line-of-duty determination. An investigating officer selected by the chain of command is appointed to conduct the investigation, if necessary. There are provisions for review of line-of-duty determinations; for example, the PEB may ask for a re-review of the decision.

Medical Evaluation Board

Any service member who is discovered to have a medical condition that calls into question his or her ability to meet medical standards for service is referred first for a complete physical examination, the results of which are submitted to an MEB. RC members not on active-duty status are referred for medical evaluation when their ability to meet medical standards comes into question. This may occur, for example, when a "medical profile" is entered in the member's record indicating a condition that limits the duties the member can perform. The MEB process is the same for all military personnel, regardless of component or active-duty status.

The MEB consists of at least two physicians from an MTF, often the MTF where the member is being treated but not always, especially for RC members not serving on active duty. On the basis of the results of the medical examination and other information, the MEB evaluates whether the member meets medical standards for continuing in service. MEB cases can result in full return to duty, limited duty for up to six months, or referral to the PEB for a determination of fitness and, in many cases, a disability evaluation. The MEB provides a narrative summary of its findings to the PEB for use in its deliberations.

In addition to the results of the medical examination, the MEB receives a report from the member's commanding officer on the performance of assigned duties, the results of any line-of-duty investigation, and information from the medical examination conducted when the member entered, if it is available.

---

2 For RC members who have accumulated at least eight years of active service, conditions are considered to be preexisting if the member becomes unfit during active service of more than 30 days.

Physical Evaluation Board

The PEB determines a member's fitness to continue in military service (i.e., whether the medical condition precludes the member from reasonably performing the duties of his or her military occupation and rank).[3] For those found unfit, the PEB assigns a disability rating by applying the Veterans Affairs Schedule for Rating Disabilities (VASRD). Only the medical conditions determined by the PEB to affect fitness are rated.

The Navy and Air Force each have a single PEB, whereas the Army has three PEBs that are assigned cases on a regional basis according to where the MEB is located. Trained personnel, generally including a physician and two line officers or civilian equivalents, adjudicate each case. The PEB conducts an initial review, termed *informal*, based on the narrative summary provided by the MEB and other relevant information, including the results of a line-of-duty investigation if there was one. Service members who do not concur with the informal board findings may request reconsideration and submit new medical information or additional supporting evidence. If found unfit, a member may request a formal PEB hearing for which he or she is allowed legal representation and can appear in person. If found unfit again, the member may petition the relevant service secretary for relief.

Physical Evaluation Board Liaison Officers (PEBLOs) are available at all MTFs to counsel service members on their legal rights and benefits during each step of the disability evaluation process. These liaison officers inform service members of the PEB's findings and help them complete an "election of options" form, indicating whether or not they accept the findings. The liaison officer then notifies the PEB about how members have decided to proceed.

The VASRD has been the basis for military DES ratings for a long time. It lists more than 700 disabilities in 14 body systems and provides evaluation criteria for each. The schedule's rating outcomes range between 0 and 100 percent, at ten-point increments, depending on severity. The last comprehensive revision of the basic VASRD occurred in 1945; in accordance with the recommendation of the 2007 Veterans Disability Benefits Commission, the VA has established a schedule for revising all sections of the VASRD over six years and for subsequent periodic updates.

In 2008, Congress mandated strict application of the VASRD, except when alternative criteria resulting in a higher rating level have been established by DoD and the VA. Prior to 2008, the PEBs had somewhat more discretion in their use of the VASRD. Also in 2008, DoD established the Physical Disability Board of Review to ensure

[3] DoD Directive 1332.18 states, "The sole standard to be used in making determinations of unfitness due to physical disability shall be unfitness to perform the duties of the member's office, grade, rank or rating because of disease or injury." The directive also specifies the requirements for medical separation and retirement. For members with less than eight years of service, the medical condition must have arisen during service after 30 days or in the line of duty during the first 30 days. Members who have more than eight years of active service are eligible for disability compensation even if the disabling condition existed prior to service. Conditions must be permanent and not the result of misconduct or neglect.

fairness by reviewing the ratings assigned to personnel who were previously found to be unfit and who received a disability rating below 30 percent. These cases initially resulted in a medical separation instead of a medical retirement, and as described below, the benefits for the two outcomes differ significantly.

Military Disability Compensation

A service member's combined disability rating for all conditions rated by the PEB determines whether he or she receives a lump-sum disability severance payment or lifelong disability retirement payments. Service members with 0-, 10-, or 20-percent disability ratings and less than 20 years' service receive a lump-sum payment upon separation from the military according to the formula:

Years of creditable service × highest monthly base pay × 2.

The largest number of enlisted personnel referred to the DES are at the rank of E-4. At 2011 base pay rates, an E-4 with four years of creditable service would receive a severance payment of about $17,000 at separation. An officer at the most common rank, O-3, with eight years of service would receive a severance payment of $83,000.

Members awarded combined disability ratings of at least 30 percent receive disability retirement compensation. The monthly benefit is the higher of two calculations, where the base-pay amount used is the average of the highest 36 months of base pay prior to discharge:

Percent disability rating × monthly base pay, or

Years of creditable service × 2.5 percent × monthly base pay.

In most cases, disability retirement pay is capped at 75 percent of the base-pay amount.[4] A rough estimate based on the pay tables for 2009–2011 shows that an E-4 who is separated in 2011 with four years of service would receive from $600 per month with a 30-percent rating to a maximum of $1,500 per month. The range for an O-3 with eight years of service is $1,550 to $3,900. These calculations use the first method above because it results in a higher amount. Relatively few of those who are medically retired benefit from the second method; an individual with a 30-percent rating has to have more than 12 years of service to benefit from the second method.

Disability retirees receive the other benefits of military retirement, including lifetime TRICARE eligibility for themselves and their dependents. Like regular retirement pay, DoD disability retirement pay is taxable unless the disability is combat-related.

[4] Members with more than 30 years of service can receive more than 75 percent. While on the Temporary Disability Retirement List (TDRL), discharged personnel receive a minimum of 50 percent times their base retirement pay.

Coordination with the VA Disability System

Any veteran can apply for VA disability benefits. The VA rates all medical conditions that it determines to be service-connected, regardless of whether or not the condition made the individual unfit for military service. Research for the Veterans' Disability Benefits Commission found that 80 percent of veterans who had received a DoD disability rating subsequently applied for VA benefits (Christensen et al., 2007). In general, the VA ratings of those veterans were higher than their DoD ratings; more conditions were reflected in the VA ratings, and the VA ratings of the same conditions were somewhat higher, on average. Unlike DoD's rating, the VA's rating is not permanent and may be adjusted over time as a veteran's condition changes.

Until recently, military personnel with a line-of-duty or service-connected disability had to navigate the DoD and VA systems sequentially, undergoing two comprehensive medical examinations. This was a time-consuming process, and as a result, eligibility for VA benefits was often not established for some time after discharge from military service. To simplify the overall process, the departments developed the Integrated Disability Evaluation System (IDES), which they piloted in 2008 and phased in at other locations in 2009–2011. The IDES involves a single medical examination and disability rating procedure for use in the DES and by the VA. The examination and rating are currently being done by VA personnel or by staff under VA contract. The results of the medical examination are submitted to an MEB, and a PEB determines whether the member is fit to continue in service. The DoD disability rating is based on the ratings established for all disabling conditions incurred or aggravated in the line of duty, and the VA rating is based on the ratings for all service-connected conditions. Under this system, consistency in the rating of individual medical conditions is ensured, but the overall DoD and VA ratings may factor in different medical conditions. Members who are medically separated or retired from service leave with their VA disability rating established and should receive any VA compensation to which they are entitled a month after separation.

DoD and the VA have established goals for the amount of time needed to complete each phase of the IDES process: 100 days for the MEB phase, 30 days for the informal PEB phase, 30 days for the formal PEB phase if there is one, and up to 60 days for appeals and to complete PEB administrative processing (Government Accountability Office, 2010). The dates recorded in the DES data provided by the services for this research cannot be used to evaluate reliably how well these goals are being achieved, but other analysis indicates that cases completed in March 2011 averaged one-third more days than the combined goals specify (Government Accountability Office, 2011).

The initial sites that piloted IDES experienced higher rates of satisfaction among service members going through the system, but processing times have been long because of staffing shortages and heavier-than-expected caseloads, along with other start-up problems (Government Accountability Office, 2010).

DoD and VA disability compensation are also coordinated. Veterans given a combined VA disability rating of 10 percent or higher receive tax-exempt monthly compensation that depends on the percent rating and, for those with a rating of 30 percent or higher, whether the veteran has a spouse and dependents. Congress authorizes the payment amounts annually. In 2011, the monthly payment is $123 for veterans with a 10-percent disability rating (with or without dependents) and $2,932 for veterans with a 100-percent disability and a spouse and one child. The VA also increases the amount provided to veterans with specific impairments through a schedule of Special Monthly Compensation payments.

In general, individuals cannot receive disability pay from both DoD and the VA. Lump-sum severance payments from DoD are offset by initial VA payments, and there is a dollar-for-dollar reduction in monthly military disability pay for individuals who also receive VA disability pay. In effect, the higher of the two amounts is paid.

There are two exceptions to the general rule that VA payments offset DoD payments: The Concurrent Retirement and Disability Payment (CRDP) program is phasing out the offset to military pay for all retired members who qualified for regular military retirement after 20 years of creditable service and have a combined VA disability rating of at least 50 percent. The phase-out, which began in 2004 and ends in 2014, eliminated 50 percent of the offset in 2007 and 94 percent in 2010. The Combat-Related Special Compensation (CRSC) program provides a special monthly payment equal to the amount of the offset to military retired pay resulting from the receipt of VA disability compensation attributable to combat-related disabilities. The payment under this program also depends on years served and retired pay base, so the amount received is less for members who were medically retired after only a few years of service.

In addition to monthly disability pay, the VA provides healthcare and other benefits. Eligibility for these benefits depends on a number of factors, including disability rating. Individuals eligible for TRICARE and VA healthcare may use either or both systems.

DES Outcomes for Fiscal Years 2007–2010

To determine whether DES outcomes for RC members differ from those for AC members, we analyzed the records of disability cases that were initiated in fiscal years 2007–2010 in the Army, Navy, and Air Force disability systems. The services provided information on all cases for which an informal board decision was made during this four-year period. The data capture the early effects of the important changes described above in the DoD and VA disability evaluation systems. Analysis of data from earlier years is available in the reports of the Veterans' Disability Benefits Commission (Veterans' Disability Benefits Commission, 2007) and the Government Accountability Office (Government Accountability Office, 2006).

The format and content of the data provided to us by the services differed. It was possible to create comparable data records for Army and Navy disability cases, but as described below, the Air Force data were more limited and required separate analysis.

The Army dataset included the final records for all cases handled by Army MEBs during 2007–2010 and the corresponding informal- and periodic-review PEB records that matched these MEB cases. There was one record for each MEB case and one for each completed informal board review and each periodic review for individuals originally put on the TDRL. A total of 54,320 individuals had both MEB and PEB records.[5] Records for 8,118 individuals who were initially put on the TDRL before FY 2007 and for whom the dataset included only periodic-review information were deleted. An additional 4,000 records were deleted because of duplicate, missing, or inconsistent data. Our final analysis file for the Army therefore consisted of 42,189 records.

The Navy data included all the individual administrative (transaction) records generated for each PEB case. The PEB records included information about the date and location of the MEB for each case. Most cases had multiple records. Using individual identifiers that were scrambled to protect individual identity, a single record was constructed for each unique case, and variables were constructed describing the informal board review, the appeal if there was one, and any periodic reviews associated with those the informal board put on the TDRL. The file contained records for 9,718 Marine Corps personnel and 10,582 Navy personnel. Of these, 2,833 were individuals for whom the only action during FY 2007–2010 was a periodic review. After deleting about 1,200 more records because of incomplete or missing information, the final Navy analysis file contained information on 16,268 individuals.

The Air Force dataset contained a single record for each individual who had a PEB decision during FY 2007–2010, for a total of 16,020 cases. The information recorded included the MEB date and location and the most recent disposition of the case. Unlike the Army and Navy files, the Air Force data files do not include complete information for each stage of the PEB process for those initially put on the TDRL. The data allow identification of individuals who were put on the TDRL after the informal review only if a subsequent periodic review had not been completed by the end of FY 2010. As we show below for the Army and Navy cases, a final disposition is unlikely to have been made for cases that entered the system in 2009–2010. Therefore, our analysis of informal outcomes for the Air Force focused on data from the most recent two years—a total of 5,399 observations.

---

[5] Almost all the MEB records that did not match a PEB record were coded ACTIVE (cases that have had an MEB initiated but have not reached PEB adjudication and disposition; these may have been stopped or terminated, were still in the MEB phase, or were forwarded to but not completed by the PEB); EPTS (medical condition determined to be existing prior to service); or IET (medical separation during initial entry training).

Descriptive statistics for all the variables used in our analysis data files are presented in Tables A.5 through A.9 in the Appendix.

DES Caseload, Disposition, and Process Time

The probability that a service member will be referred to the DES varies widely across the services and across components within the services. Table 3.1 compares the number of disability cases per 1,000 members in each service and component, focusing on those who have been deployed at least once since 2001. The rates were calculated by dividing the number of FY 2009 disability cases for AC and RC members with deployment experience by the total number of AC and RC members serving at the end of FY 2008. The calculations show that Army personnel are at least twice as likely to be referred as personnel in the other services. Referral for RC members is only about one-third as frequent as it is for active-duty members of the same service.

To further explore the difference in the rates of DES referral of AC and RC members, we compared the distributions of VASRD codes for AC and RC members by service and by whether the member has been deployed since 2001. A complete listing is given in Table A.4 in the Appendix. For members who have not been deployed, the most common codes account for about the same fraction in the AC and RC; one exception is spinal conditions, which are more heavily represented among RC members. The AC-RC differences are somewhat more pronounced for members who have been deployed. In particular, RC members are more likely to have conditions linked to combat exposure, such as PTSD, major depression, anxiety disorder, and traumatic brain injury; the frequency of these conditions is one-quarter to one-half higher for RC members than for AC members, and it is twice as high in the Air Force. Research

Table 3.1
Disability Cases per 1,000 Service Members Deployed Since 2001, FY 2009

	Active	Guard/Reserve
All cases		
Army	17.7	5.4
Navy	7.4	2.8
Marine Corps	9.3	2.5
Air Force	15.0	5.4
Cases involving PTSD (all services)	3.0	1.4

shows that the incidence for Guard/Reserve members who have deployed is at least as high as it is for active-duty members.[6] Therefore, the fraction of RC members referred to the DES who have a diagnosis of PTSD in Table 3.1 should be considerably higher, but instead, as the last row in the table shows, the number of RC disability cases involving PTSD is half that of AC cases.

What are some possible explanations for the differences in disability referral rates? Unlike other disability systems (including the VA system), members do not apply to the DoD disability system. They are referred by a medical provider or at the initiative of their unit. RC members are less likely to be in treatment by a military provider who is trained to identify individuals with potentially duty-limiting medical conditions. These conditions thus may be less likely to be identified by their units or civilian providers. Alternatively, members who believe they may have a compensable medical condition may ask for a referral, but RC members may be less likely to seek a referral, for several reasons. They may be deterred by the requirement for a line-of-duty decision. If they want to remain in service, RC members may find it easier to perform the more limited duties of part-time service when they are not activated. Also, an in-depth analysis may show that these simple statistics are misleading.[7]

The Army has by far the largest number of disability cases (Table 3.2). Few of those who formally enter the DES and are referred to a PEB receive a disability disposition other than separation or retirement. This is not surprising, because the MEB should identify most individuals whose medical condition does not preclude their continuing to serve. Also, few cases end in a separation without benefits. Benefits are denied only to those who were found unfit for duty by the PEB because of a medical condition that was ruled not in the line of duty, a result of negligence or misconduct, or for another specified reason. For our analysis of DES outcomes, the few cases that did not result in a disability separation or retirement were omitted.

Informal PEB Disposition

Figure 3.2 shows the informal PEB result for cases that ended in a disability separation or retirement. Since 2007, the fraction of cases resulting in separation has decreased, probably because of the criticisms of DES outcomes described above and the congressional directives on rating practices. The IDES system was piloted and expanded during the same time period, but only 13 percent of the cases in FY 2007–2010 were in IDES. Therefore, it is unlikely that the change in disposition observed over this time period was the result of IDES.

---

[6] In a 2007–2008 survey of previously deployed military personnel and veterans, RC respondents were twice as likely to report symptoms of PTSD (Adamson et al., 2008). The 95-percent confidence interval for this estimate is large, but the difference is statistically significant at the 0.05 level. This result is consistent with the results of other studies of PTSD prevalence.

[7] An in-depth analysis would require the collection of medical records for RC members, a difficult undertaking.

Table 3.2
Number and Initial Disposition of Cases: Army and Navy PEBs, Cases Initiated in FY 2007–2010

Fiscal Year	Total	Disability Separation or Retirement	Non-Disability Separation	Fit, Limited Duty, or Other Outcome
		Army		
2007	10,564	9,233	473	858
2008	11,523	10,328	247	948
2009	12,446	11,306	126	1,014
2010[a]	7,656	7,018	68	570
Total	42,189	37,885	914	3,390
		Navy and Marine Corps		
2007	4,843	3,154	473	1,216
2008	4,745	3,467	377	901
2009	4,414	3,319	330	765
2010[a]	2,266	1,655	174	437
Total	16,268	11,595	1,354	3,319
		Air Force		
2009	3,128	2,207	94	827
2010[a]	2,271	1,723	106	442
Total	5,399	3,930	200	1,269

[a] Excludes cases with no informal PEB decision.

Individuals initially placed on the TDRL are reexamined after they have been on the list for 18 to 24 months; those with a diagnosis of PTSD are reexamined for that condition after six months and again after 18 to 24 months for any other medical conditions. All TDRL cases must receive a final disposition after five years on the list. The Army and Navy data were adequate for tracking TDRL cases over time, but the Air Force data were not. Just over half of the Army and Navy cases that entered the DES in 2007 had received a final disposition by the end of 2010 (Figure 3.3). In the 2008 DES cohort, only 30 percent were resolved by 2010, and very few entering after 2008 had a final disposition.

Eighty-four percent of the TDRL cases in our dataset that had a final disposition were put on the permanent retirement list (Figure 3.3). However, it is unlikely that the one-half of FY 2007 TDRL cases that were resolved were representative of all TDRL cases in that year. Those that were resolved may have been more or less serious than

Figure 3.2
Initial Disposition of Cases Ending in a Disability Separation or Retirement, by Fiscal Year

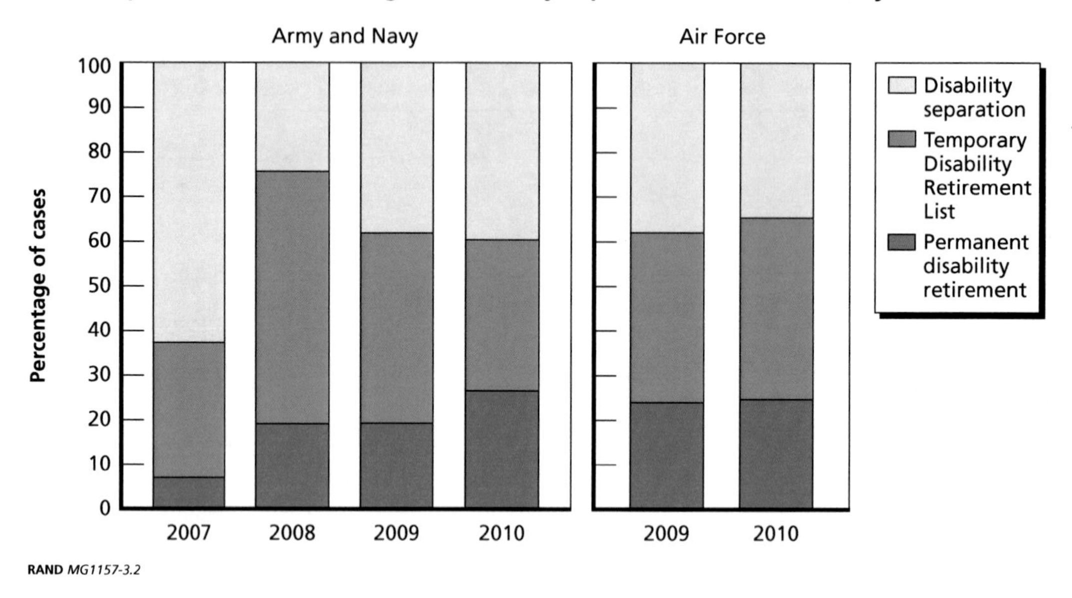

RAND *MG1157-3.2*

Figure 3.3
Status of Army and Navy 2007–2008 TDRL Cases at the End of FY 2010

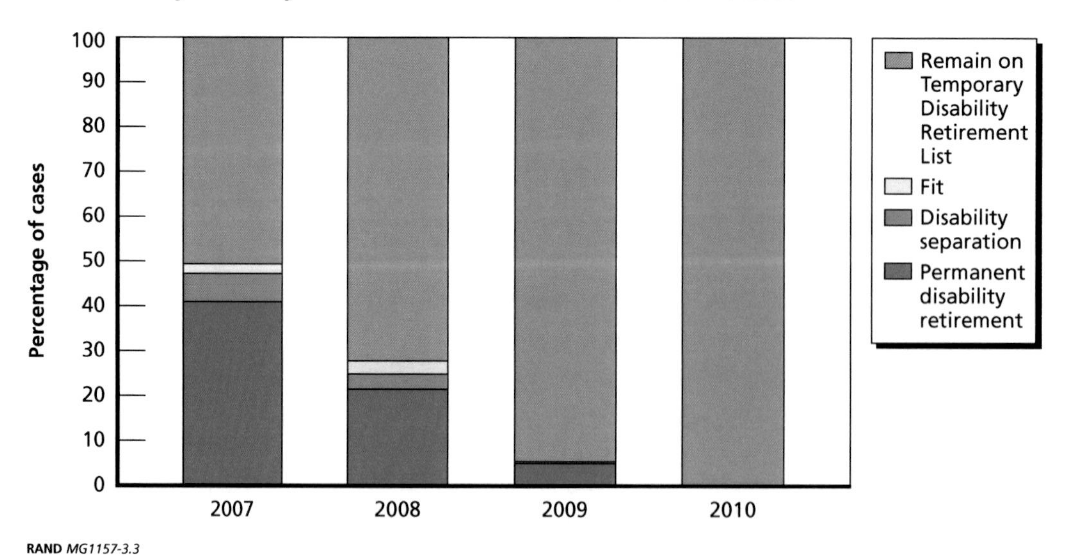

RAND *MG1157-3.3*

those that were not resolved until after FY 2010. A review of the final disposition of all cases put on the TDRL in 2000–2003 found that three-fifths of them ended up on the Permanent Disability Retirement List (PDRL), one-quarter had their disability rating lowered and received a disability separation, and most of the remainder were separated without benefits (Government Accountability Office, 2009). At the same time, a DoD report to Congress on the TDRL concluded that the purpose of the list has shifted over time from maximizing the number of injured or ill service members who can return to duty to allowing more time for recovery before a final disability determination is made (Office of the Under Secretary of Defense [Personnel and Readiness], 2008). DoD reported that half of all the TDRL cases from 2000 to 2007 with a final disposition had the same final rating they received initially, 39 percent received a lower final rating, and 11 percent received a higher final rating. The same report found that almost three in five of the TDRL cases from 2000–2002, all of which had been finalized, ended up as permanent disability retirements. However, the report indicated that of the 2005 cases finalized by the end of 2007, a higher fraction (two-thirds) ended up on the PDRL. Given how long it takes to resolve TDRL cases, it is not possible to determine whether the higher completion rate of TDRL cases from 2007–2008 in the dataset used for this study represents a shift in final disposition or an increased ability in recent years to resolve permanent disability retirement cases. It is too early to tell whether the shift in disability rating policy that occurred in 2008 will affect the final disposition of TDRL cases and lead to more disability retirements.

The data show that, as policy requires, essentially all PTSD cases referred to the DES in 2009 and 2010 were put on the TDRL; this was also true for almost all the PTSD cases in 2007 and 2008. After the policy memo directing a minimum temporary rating of 50 percent, the ratings for cases involving PTSD increased in 2009 and 2010 to a minimum of 50 percent in every service. Since the disposition of PTSD cases, especially in more recent years, has been uniform for RC and AC members, those cases are excluded from the analysis of informal PEB disposition below. However, the cases are retained in the analysis of the informal PEB rating percentage.

DES Process Times

The average number of days to complete the MEB and PEB phases of the DES is shown in Figure 3.4 for Army and Navy cases. The figure does not include cases that involved an appeal of an informal PEB decision or a formal PEB hearing; on average, across the services, these cases take about 70 days longer than cases that are not appealed. As discussed above, DES dates are likely to be captured differently in the service DES data systems. The Army data are the most accurate, and they show the longest average times to complete both the MEB and PEB phases of the DES. The Navy legacy system data records the date the physician's MEB referral was entered into the administrative record. This may have occurred some time after the referral was actually initiated. The Navy now records the date the physician signs the MEB referral for IDES cases. The Air Force provided the date the narrative summary of the MEB review was received by the PEB, not the date the case was referred to the MEB.

The processing time for an individual case depends on the complexity of the case and the completeness and quality of the information provided for adjudication. It also depends on how well the services resource their processes, given their workloads. The

Figure 3.4
Mean Number of Days for MEB and Informal PEB: Army and Navy Cases Initiated in FY 2007–2010

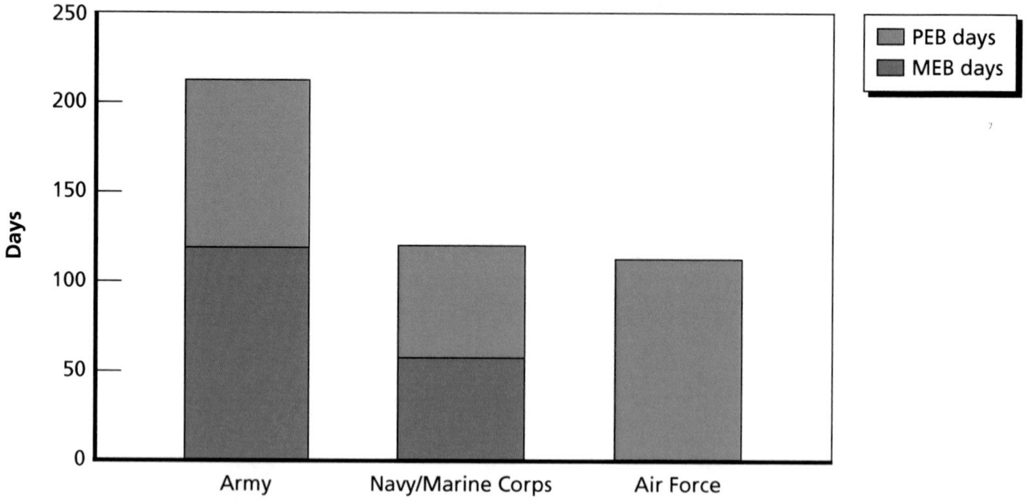

NOTE: Air Force MEB days not available.
RAND *MG1157-3.4*

service differences shown here reflect the resources devoted to the DES process, relative to the service's disability workload.

Differences in Outcomes for RC and AC Personnel

To estimate the differences in DES outcomes between AC and RC personnel, we used regression analysis, controlling for the medical condition as represented by the VASRD codes, the military service, and the fiscal year the case entered the DES. The data included up to four VASRD codes that were in the PEB rating. Half of the Army and Navy cases were coded with a nonspecific DoD-unique code for musculoskeletal or muscle condition, and these are captured by three broad codes. We combined less common diagnoses by type of condition, as shown in the Appendix. Since the VASRD codes do not fully describe the medical information available to the PEB for rating, the regressions included variables for individual characteristics that might be expected to convey additional information about the individual's health condition: age, gender, and military occupation.[8] Marital status and rank (enlisted versus officer) were also included as covariates, but in general, they were not statistically significant.

---

[8] If military occupation is strongly correlated with component status, it could be difficult to separately identify the effects of RC status from the effects of occupation. There are some differences in the distribution of military occupation between components. AC members in the DES are more likely to be in a combat occupation. The most significant differences are the following: 29 percent of AC members are in the infantry, gun crew, seaman-

The regressions model provides three outcomes: informal PEB disposition, informal percentage rating, and processing time (MEB and informal PEB time modeled separately). The analysis focuses on informal PEB outcomes, because so few of the cases in our dataset had final outcomes, and, as discussed above, final outcomes are highly correlated with initial outcomes. Separate analyses were conducted on the combined Army and Navy DES data for all years (FY 2007–2010) and on Air Force data for 2009–2010 only.[9] In light of the more limited time period and smaller sample size for the Air Force analyses, this discussion emphasizes the Army and Navy results and summarizes any differences in the results for the Air Force separately.

Informal board disposition is analyzed with a multinomial probit to account for separation, PDRL, and TDRL. We employed ordinary least squares (OLS) estimation for the informal board rating (0 to 100 percent) and (log) MEB and PEB process times. The MEB and PEB time data are distributed with a long tail that fits a lognormal distribution. Detailed results including coefficients and standard errors for the explanatory variables in each equation are provided in the Appendix.

DES Outcomes for the Army and Navy

Informal PEB Disposition. Figure 3.5 shows selected regression results for Army and Navy informal PEB disposition. Panel a plots the difference in the percentage of cases receiving a permanent disability retirement, temporary disability retirement, or disability separation in each service. Panels b and c show results for other member characteristics and the year and type of DES (IDES or legacy) and for selected VASRD codes related to deployment, respectively. The charts in the first two panels employ the same scale to facilitate comparison, but the scale in the third panel is different to account for the larger differences in outcomes across medical conditions.

There are only modest differences in disposition between RC and AC members after the diagnoses recorded by the VASRD codes are controlled for. RC members are slightly more likely to receive a temporary disability retirement than a permanent disability retirement, and Navy personnel are somewhat more likely to receive a disability separation.

The differences between AC and RC are small relative to the shift in the types of decisions over time, as illustrated by the differences between FY 2009 and FY 2007 in panel b of Figure 3.5. Further analysis shows that the Army accounts for most of the change in dispositions in recent years. The early IDES cases in our dataset are also somewhat more likely to result in a permanent retirement decision, but the difference

---

ship occupation versus 18 percent in the RC, and 11 percent of AC members are in communications and intelligence versus 5 percent of RC members. These differences should not pose a problem for the estimation of the RC-AC difference.

[9] Separate analyses of the Army and Navy data revealed few differences, so only the combined results are reported.

Figure 3.5
Differences in the Probability of Informal PEB Dispositions: Army and Navy Cases Initiated in FY 2007–2010

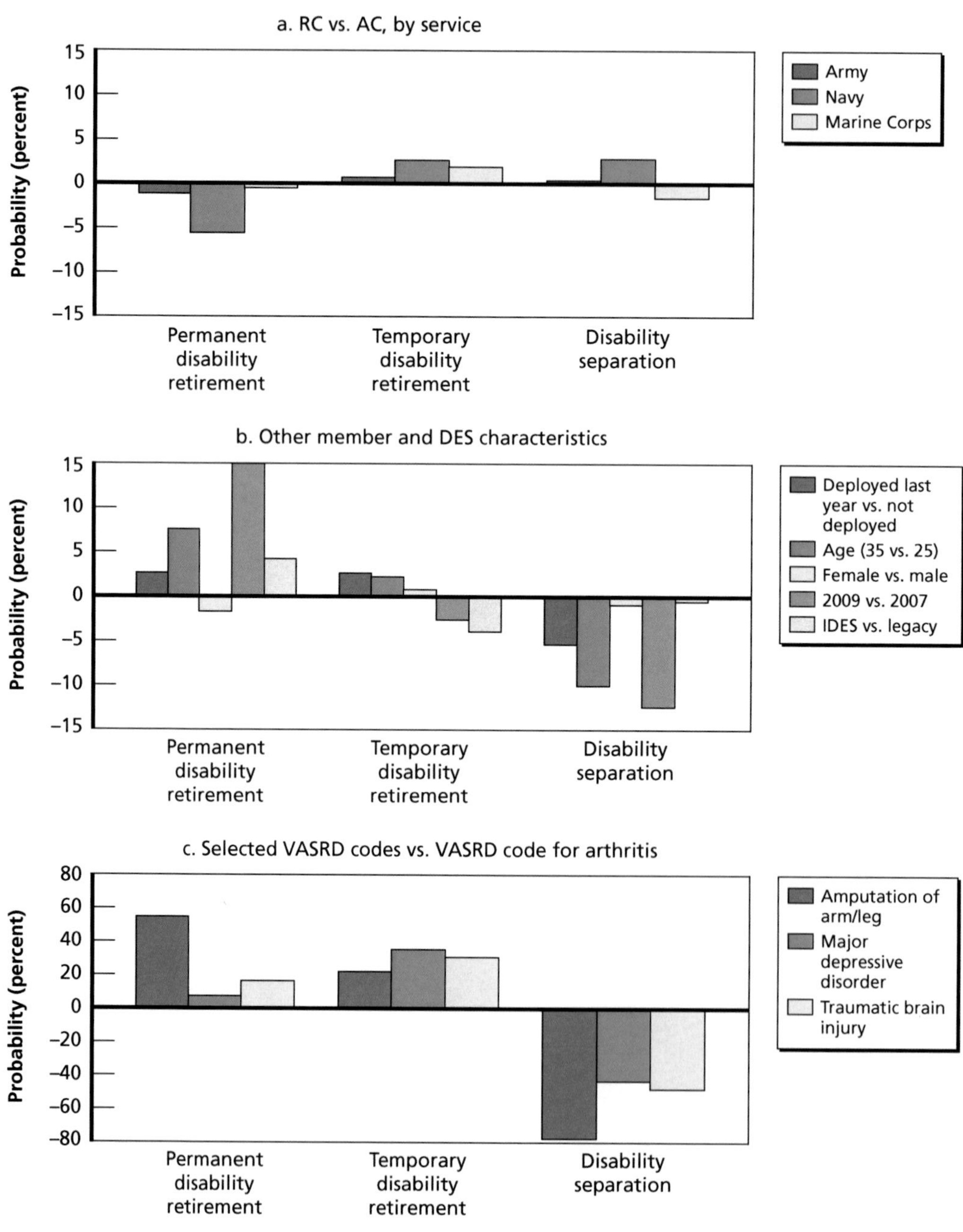

RAND *MG1157-3.5*

is small. Retirement decisions are more common among older members and those who have been deployed. It is not surprising to find that older members present with disabilities that are more likely to exceed the 30-percent rating threshold for a disability retirement. Panel b compares the dispositions for members deployed within a year of being referred to the DES and those who have not been deployed since 2001. Cases arising soon after deployment may be more likely to be combat-related and to differ in unobserved ways in the medical conditions documented. However, the more complete results in the Appendix do not support a conclusion that outcomes differ with the timing of DES entry after deployment.

As expected, the differences in outcomes attributed to VASRD codes are sizable compared with differences attributed to individual characteristics. Panel c compares outcomes for cases with selected VASRD codes associated with the current conflict, compared with a common condition, arthritis, which is associated with a low probability of retirement. Recall that PTSD cases were omitted from this analysis because their outcomes became deterministic in FY 2009.

Disability Rating. Analysis of disability ratings reveals a modest, positive difference in ratings between RC members and AC members in the Army and Navy/Marine Corps (Figure 3.6). Compared with the mean rating for the Army and Navy/Marine Corps of 32.7 [10] and the difference in ratings across VASRD codes in panel c of Figure 3.6, the differences shown in panel b by type of DES system, service, deployment history, and age are also modest.

DES Process Time. To estimate DES process time, separate regressions were run for the Army and Navy disability systems because of the substantial difference in mean times shown in Figure 3.4 and the Government Accountability Office audit cited earlier that found differences in how the PEBs record processing dates. Cases involving an appeal of the informal PEB decision or a formal PEB hearing are not included in this analysis. The results provide estimates of the percentage change in the number of days to complete the MEB and PEB phases of the DES associated with each of the explanatory variables. Controlling for VASRD codes and other individual and system characteristics, there are differences between AC and RC process times in both services (Figure 3.7). Process times for Army RC disability cases are shorter, whereas the opposite is true for the Navy and Marine Corps. The differences are more pronounced at the PEB phase than they are at the MEB phase.

Process times—DES process times, in particular—are longer in more recent years, and the IDES is taking longer in the Army system but not in the Navy system.[11]

---

[10] The average informal board rating for cases initiated in FY 2007–2010 was 33.0 for the Army and 31.6 for the Navy/Marine Corps. The ratings in the Air Force data for the same years averaged 32.9; the vast majority of these are informal board ratings, but some reflect changes made after a periodic reexamination.

[11] The Government Accountability Office (2011) also found that the IDES system has been taking longer in recent years.

Figure 3.6
Difference in Informal PEB Ratings: Army and Navy Cases Initiated in FY 2007–2010

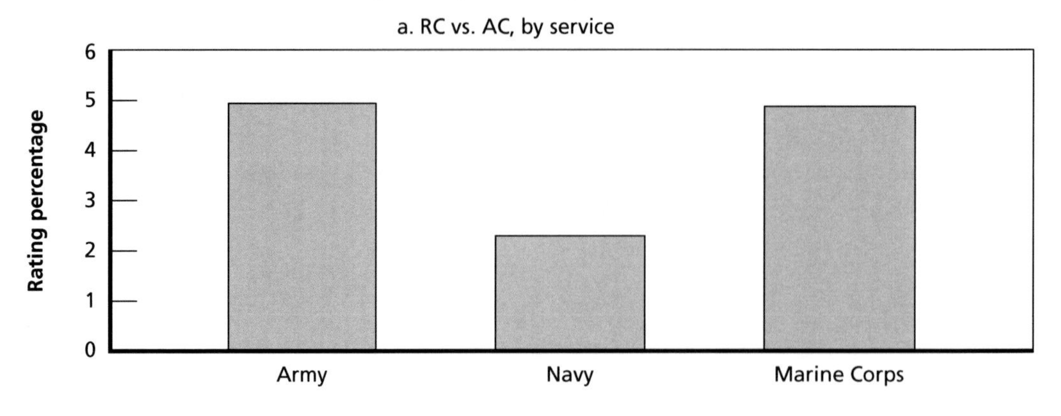

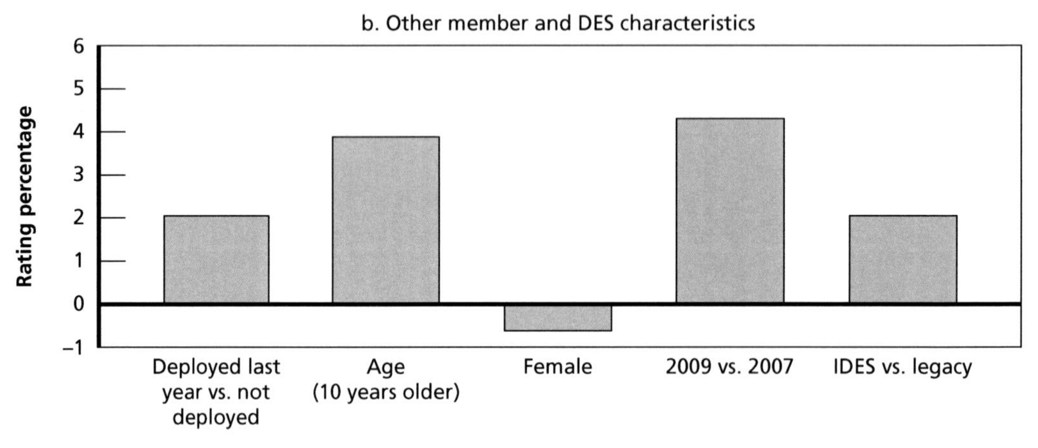

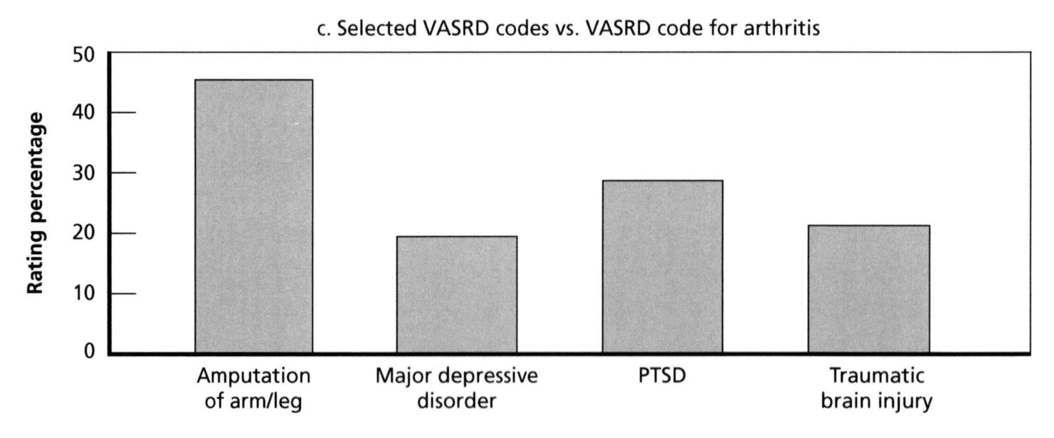

RAND *MG1157-3.6*

Figure 3.7
Difference in DES Processing Time: Army and Navy Cases Initiated in FY 2007–2010 with No Appeal or Formal PEB

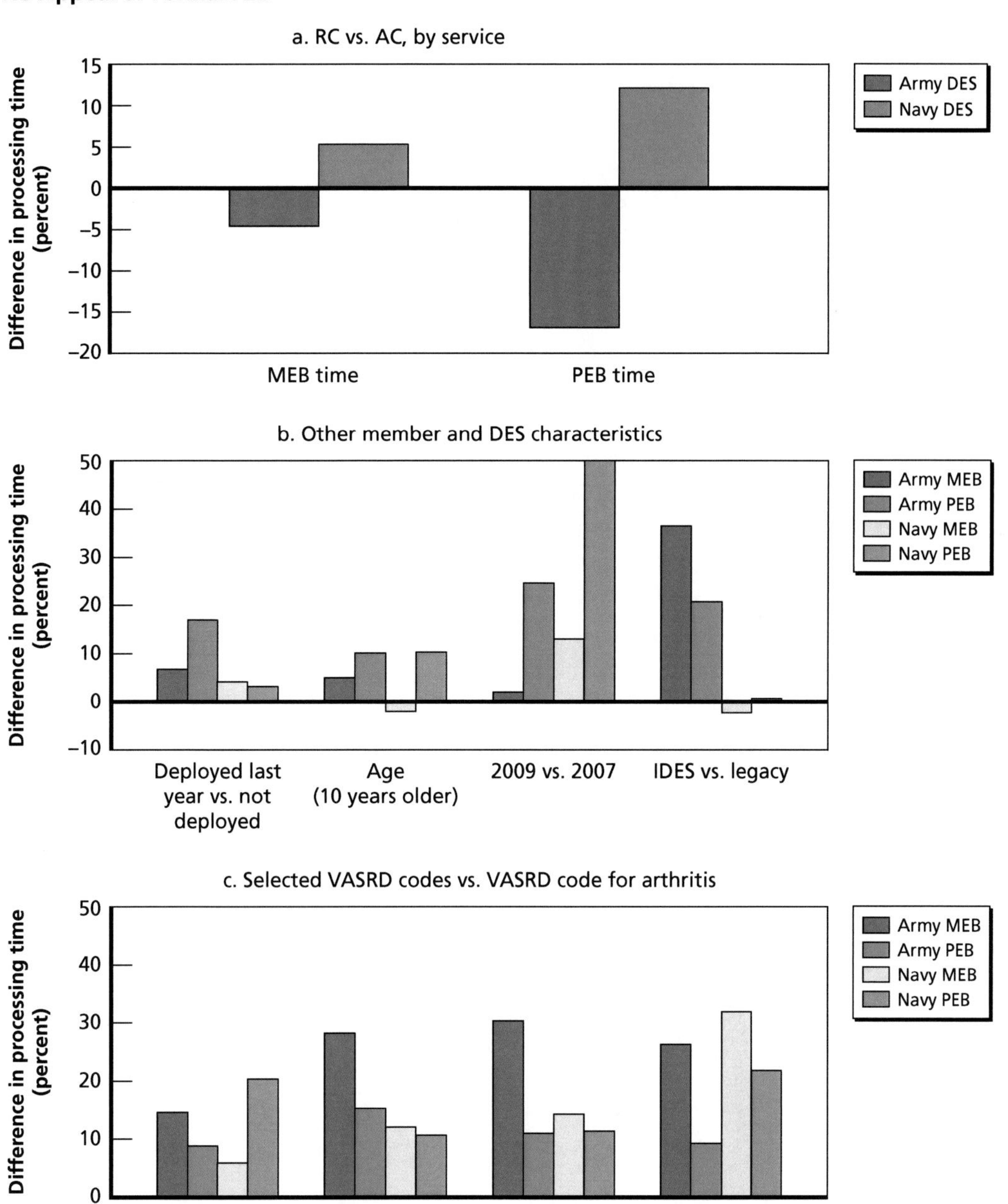

RAND *MG1157-3.7*

Consistent with the hypothesis advanced earlier that older members present more-complex cases, the process time for older members is slightly longer. Finally, the time to evaluate cases for members who have been deployed is somewhat longer overall (panel b), and cases involving a war-related condition take longer than cases involving a more routine condition such as arthritis (panel c).

Within a service, MEB times vary considerably depending on which MTF handles the medical evaluation (these results are given in the Appendix). The regression analysis controls for this variation, so the RC-AC difference in MEB time is not driven by the members' geographic locations.

DES Outcomes for the Air Force

For our analysis, we used Air Force data for FY 2009–2010. To apply the multinomial probit method to estimate the regression for informal PEB disposition (PDRL, TDRL, disability separation), the smaller Air Force sample size dictated the use of fewer explanatory variables. Indicator variables that were not statistically significant in our initial Air Force analysis using other methods—for officer, deployment more than two years prior to DES entry, and occupation—were omitted. The VASRD code indicators were combined based on the preliminary results, as described in the Appendix. The variables in the analysis of disability rating and PEB time were unchanged; MEB time was not included in the analysis because the data contain only a measure of the time to forward the MEB results to the PEB.

Figure 3.8 shows the estimated RC-AC difference in disposition and PEB time for the Air Force; not shown is the difference in the percentage rating, which was small (one percentage point) and not statistically significant. The results indicate that RC members in the Air Force are less likely to be put on the PDRL by the informal board and more likely to be separated or put on the TDRL. Overall, Air Force RC members received a slightly lower disability rating during the two years analyzed. These results should be viewed with caution, however, given the limited sample size.[12] In the raw data, unadjusted for the condition(s) rated, Air Force RC members were less likely to go on the PDRL and more likely to get a TDRL or separation decision. More data are needed to obtain a reliable picture of disability dispositions in the Air Force.

Summary

As with healthcare, the major difference in the treatment of RC members and AC members in disability evaluation results from the line-of-duty requirement. AC mem-

---

[12] Results using a logit specification (one equation for retirement—PDRL or TDRL—versus separation and another for PDRL versus TDRL, conditional on being retired) were similar. Although this logit specification does not allow for joint estimation of all three outcomes, it produced similar results for all the services and could be estimated using all variables with the Air Force data. Therefore, limiting the variable list in the multinomial probit specification does not appear to affect the results.

Figure 3.8
Differences in DES Outcomes: Air Force Cases Initiated in FY 2009–2010

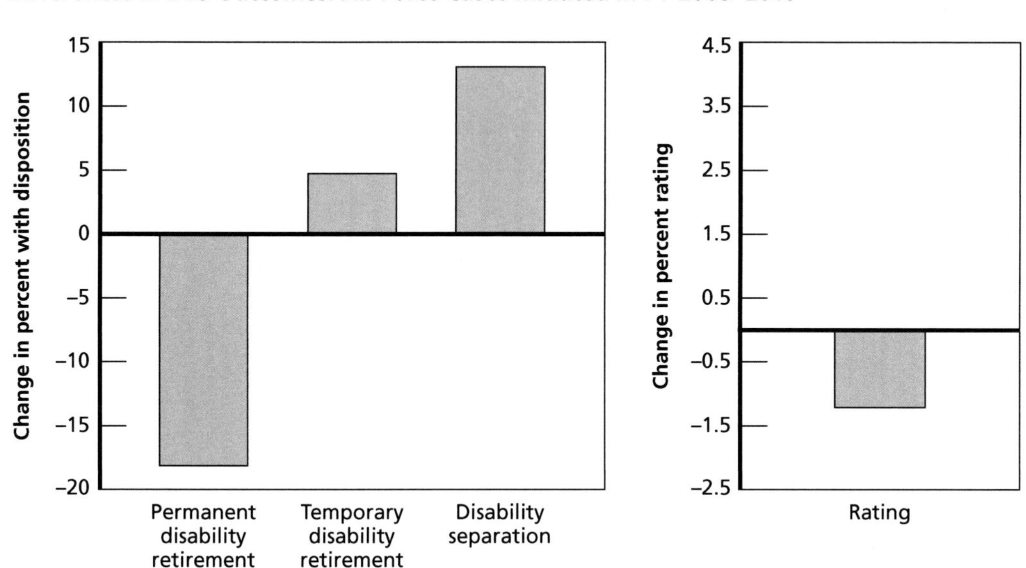

RAND *MG1157-3.8*

bers are considered to be continuously on duty, so the health problems that arise while they are in service are almost always a basis for disability benefits. RC members are not covered for disabilities that are not incurred or aggravated as a result of training or active service. Moreover, they are only approximately one-third as likely to be referred to the DES. As expected, given this difference, war-related medical conditions are more common among RC members, but it is not possible to conclude from the data available for this study whether all RC members with line-of-duty conditions are identified and evaluated for disability. The rates of referral for PTSD for service members who have deployed since 2001 suggest that some RC members may be missed.

Once referred for disability evaluation, the process is the same across components, and there is little difference between RC and AC dispositions. For those with PTSD, the strict policy guidance of TDRL placement ensures equal outcomes. For others, once the medical condition captured by the VASRD code is controlled for, the differences are at most only a few percentage points.

CHAPTER FOUR

Conclusion

The important operational role the RC has assumed since 2001 raises questions about the structure of RC compensation and benefits, including the benefits provided through DoD health and disability programs. The research reported here supports consideration of this issue by the 11th QRMC. The major findings are:

- Thirty percent of RC members lack health insurance to cover care for non–service-related conditions. The TRS program offers the option of purchasing health insurance through the military on terms that compare favorably with typical employer benefits. Although an increasing number of eligible members are enrolling in TRS, the program does not appear to be effectively targeting those most likely to be uninsured.
- Health reform would be expected to decrease the fraction of uninsured to 11 percent in the absence of TRS. However, TRS costs will compare favorably with the new options available with health reform (PPACA), so the individual mandate is likely to increase TRS enrollment.
- RC members are referred to the DES at one-third the rate of AC members, at least in part because those who are not serving full-time on active duty have more difficulty meeting the line-of-duty requirement. However, DES referral rates for PTSD for previously deployed RC members are also lower despite evidence that the incidence of PTSD is at least as high in the RC.
- RC members referred for disability evaluation receive dispositions (and thus benefits) that are similar to those for AC members referred to the DES. The times to complete the MEB and informal PEB steps in the process are also similar.

These findings suggest that DoD may want to consider ways to better coordinate TRS with other insurance options that will be available to RC members and that the identification of RC members who experience health consequences from deployment leading to disability merits further investigation.

APPENDIX

Variable Definitions, Descriptive Statistics, and Detailed Regression Results

Table A.1
Health Insurance Regressions: Variable Means

Variable	Unweighted Mean	Weighted Mean
Have Medical Insurance or Had Insurance Before Current Deployment	0.7964	0.6975
Army National Guard	0.1796	0.4348
Army Reserve	0.2037	0.2578
Navy Reserve	0.1921	0.0860
Marine Corps Reserve	0.1378	0.0534
Air National Guard	0.1191	0.0966
Air Reserve (omitted)	0.1677	0.0714
Female	0.1991	0.1866
E-1–E-3	0.0740	0.1677
E-4	0.1509	0.2733
E-5–E-6	0.1895	0.3081
E-7–E-9	0.0647	0.0940
Officers (omitted)	0.5209	0.1569
Never Married	0.2633	0.3965
Previously Married	0.1201	0.1343
Married (omitted)	0.6166	0.4770
Non-Hispanic Black	0.0962	0.1361
Hispanic	0.1113	0.1265

Table A.1—Continued

Variable	Unweighted Mean	Weighted Mean
Non-Hispanic White/Other (omitted)	0.7925	0.7374
No Children under 23	0.4404	0.5243
Part-Time Employed	0.1300	0.1773
Not Employed (for Pay)	0.3542	0.4239
Full-Time Employed (omitted)	0.5158	0.3988
Full-Time Student	0.1384	0.2234
Part-Time Student	0.0984	0.0995
Not Student (omitted)	0.7632	0.6771
Private/Public Employer	0.3554	0.3439
Self/Family Employment	0.0573	0.0512
Firm Has	0.0717	0.0820
No College	0.0745	0.1736
Some College	0.3167	0.5186
Bachelors Degree	0.3289	0.1994
Graduate Degree (omitted)	0.3544	0.2820

Table A.2
Health Insurance Regressions: Coefficients and Standard Errors

Variable	Coefficient	Standard Error
Intercept	1.01370	0.01403
Army National Guard	−0.06015	0.01475
Army Reserve	−0.02213	0.01413
Navy Reserve	−0.01419	0.01432
Marine Corps Reserve	−0.04369	0.01595
Air National Guard	0.02790	0.01618
Female	0.03420	0.01114
E-1–E-3	−0.07405	0.02216
E-4	−0.11917	0.01751
E-5–E-6	−0.05329	0.01515
E-7–E-9	0.02954	0.01980
Never Married	−0.08816	0.01286
Previously Married	−0.05286	0.01370
Non-Hispanic Black	−0.06373	0.01490
Hispanic	−0.08465	0.01373
No Children under 23	−0.02204	0.01037
Part-Time Employed	−0.13385	0.01443
Not Employed (for Pay)	−0.16566	0.01025
Private/Public Employer	−0.00331	0.00977
Self/Family Employment	0.02157	0.02350
Firm Size 1–49	−0.06377	0.01636
Full-Time Student	0.01515	0.01357
Part-Time Student	0.01129	0.01455
No College	−0.12041	0.02212
Some College	−0.05829	0.01627
Bachelors Degree	−0.02657	0.01131

Table A.3
Categorization of VASRD Codes for Regression Analysis

	VASRD Category	VASRD Codes	Number of Observations	AF Multinomial Probit Variable
1	DoD-specific code musculoskeletal disease	5099	6,494	1
2	DoD-specific code musculoskeletal injury	5199	4,708	1
3	DoD-specific code musculoskeletal injury	5299	532	1
4	Anxiety disorder	9412–9413	800	5
5	Arthritis	5002–5010	1,352	—
6	Asthma	6602	861	6
7	Bipolar disorder	9432	812	6
8	Cardiovascular condition	7000–7199	715	4
9	Digestive condition	7200–7399	879	5
10	Endocrine condition	7900–7999	603	3
11	Epilepsy	8910–8999	665	5
12	Extremity amputation or loss	5104–5125, 5160–5199	516	—[a]
13	GYN condition	7610–7699	115	6
14	Genitourinary condition	7500–7599	360	
15	Hemic condition	7700–7799	174	6
16	Infectious disease	6300–6399	157	5
17	Major depressive disorder	9434	1,428	6
18	Muscle injury	5301–5399	446	3
19	Other		133	6
20	Other mental disorder	Other codes 9201–9299, 9400–9521	582	5
21	Other musculoskeletal injury	Other codes 5100–5299	1,246	4
22	Other musculoskeletal disease	Other codes 5000–5099	3,886	2
23	Other neurological condition	Other codes 8000–8799	3,232	4
24	Other respiratory condition	6502–6899	541	4
25	Other spinal injury		783	2
26	PTSD	9411	7,370	—
27	Schizophrenia	9201–9299	617	8
28	Sense organ condition	6000–6299	608	4
29	Skin condition	7800–7899	433	4
30	Lumbosacral or cervical strain	5237	2,366	3
31	Spinal fusion	5241	1,188	5
32	Degenerative arthritis	5242	1,667	2
33	Intervertebral disc syndrome	5243	1,711	3
34	Traumatic brain injury (TBI)	8045	1,206	7

[a] Insufficient number of cases for analysis.

Table A.4
Distribution of VASRD Codes in the AC and RC

	Percentage of Cases with Code			
	Deployed Since 2001		Not Deployed Since 2001	
VASRD Category	**AC**	**RC**	**AC**	**RC**
DoD-specific code musculoskeletal disease	22.6	23.6	16.8	21.1
DoD-specific code musculoskeletal injury	15.5	19.6	10.4	12.6
DoD-specific code musculoskeletal injury	2.2	1.5	1.3	1.3
Anxiety disorder	0.9	1.3	2.7	3.5
Arthritis	9.8	10.5	7.3	11.3
Asthma	2.5	1.6	2.3	1.2
Bipolar disorder	2.5	1.5	1.8	0.9
Cardiovascular condition	1.8	2.9	1.7	2.7
Digestive condition	2.8	2.0	2.4	2.1
Endocrine condition	1.7	2.1	1.5	1.5
Epilepsy	2.4	1.2	1.6	0.8
Extremity amputation or loss	0.3	0.3	2.0	1.3
GYN condition	0.4	0.3	0.3	0.2
Genitourinary condition	1.2	1.1	1.1	1.1
Hemic condition	0.5	0.7	0.4	0.4
Infectious disease	0.5	0.6	0.3	0.2
Major depressive disorder	3.5	4.8	3.5	5.5
Muscle injury	1.5	1.0	2.5	2.1
Other	0.6	1.0	1.1	1.2
Other mental disorder	1.7	1.5	1.5	2.2
Other musculoskeletal injury	5.8	5.8	2.8	4.7
Other musculoskeletal disease	15.2	16.0	11.9	11.6
Other neurological condition	11.6	11.6	12.7	15.6
Other respiratory condition	1.2	1.9	1.6	2.3
Other spinal injury	2.3	2.7	2.6	2.2
PTSD	1.5	3.0	26.1	34.9
Schizophrenia	1.8	0.6	1.2	0.8
Sense organ condition	1.4	1.2	2.8	2.7
Skin condition	1.2	0.9	2.8	1.7
Lumbosacral or cervical strain	6.8	7.8	7.5	11.7
Spinal fusion	2.5	5.5	3.2	7.6
Degenerative arthritis	4.5	8.3	6.4	12.1
Intervertebral disc syndrome	4.0	6.3	5.8	9.2
Traumatic brain injury (TBI)	1.2	1.5	8.4	10.4

Table A.5
Disability Regressions: Sample Size and Variable Means, by Service

Variable	Army	Navy	Marine Corps	Air Force
No. of observations	37,885	5,386	6,212	3,730
FY07	0.2438	0.2900	0.2567	0.2917
FY08	0.2726	0.2991	0.2988	0.2658
FY09	0.2984	0.2746	0.2962	0.2485
FY10	0.1852	0.1363	0.1483	0.1940
Age_yrs	29.274	28.685	24.560	30.382
Female	0.1758	0.2351	0.0893	0.3217
Reserve_comp	0.1989	0.0921	0.1141	0.1438
Officer	0.0339	0.0509	0.0179	0.0714
Married	0.6344	0.5752	0.4910	0.6172
Appeal	0.0974	0.2490	0.2635	0.2081
IDES	0.1347	0.1896	0.2457	0.0472
Not Deployed Since 2001	0.3652	0.5357	0.4691	0.5288
Deployed within 1 year of MEB	0.2523	0.0900	0.1515	0.0840
Deployed within 1-2 years of MEB	0.2076	0.1281	0.1892	0.1256
Deployed within 2-3 years of MEB	0.0878	0.0863	0.0998	0.0880
Deployed within 3-4 years of MEB	0.0476	0.0583	0.0465	0.0642
Deployed 4+ years before MEB	0.0395	0.1016	0.0439	0.1094
Infantry, Gun Crews, Seamanship	0.2644	0.1134	0.3445	0.1231
Electronic Equip Repairers	0.0454	0.1285	0.0457	0.0647
Communications, Intelligence	0.0974	0.0561	0.0600	0.0694
Health Care Specialists	0.0801	0.0945	0.0182	0.0795
Other Technical & Allied Specialists	0.0281	0.0115	0.1082	0.0390
Functional Support & Admin	0.1119	0.0993	0.1151	0.1846
Electrical/Mechanical Equipment Repairers	0.1176	0.2724	0.0201	0.1906
Craftsworkers	0.0305	0.0646	0.0963	0.0436
Service and Supply Handlers	0.1658	0.0917	0.1698	0.0816
Non-Occupational	0.0167	0.0147	0.0061	0.0516
Tactical Operations Officers	0.0115	0.0130	0.0006	0.0181
Intelligence Officers	0.0026	0.0022	0.0023	0.0032
Engineering & Maint Officers	0.0054	0.0087	0.0008	0.0066
Scientists and Professionals	0.0021	0.0046	0.0000	0.0047
Health Care Officers	0.0060	0.0110	0.0014	0.0231
Administrators	0.0037	0.0054	0.0026	0.0054
Supply, Procurement Officers	0.0047	0.0041	0.0064	0.0068

Table A.5—Continued

Variable	Army	Navy	Marine Corps	Air Force
Non-occupational	0.0044	0.0026	0.0064	0.0033
DoD-unique musculoskeletal diseases	0.2198	0.0960	0.1386	0.0521
DoD-unique musculoskeletal injuries	0.1346	0.1001	0.1248	0.0259
DOD-unique muscle injuries	0.0160	0.0137	0.0167	0.0086
Anxiety disorder	0.0242	0.0154	0.0064	0.0172
Arthritis	0.0547	0.1643	0.2226	0.1039
Asthma	0.0243	0.0134	0.0142	0.0751
Bipolar disorder	0.0150	0.0444	0.0206	0.0321
Cardiovascular condition	0.0186	0.0290	0.0142	0.0397
Digestive condition	0.0195	0.0590	0.0243	0.0495
Endocrine condition	0.0146	0.0301	0.0122	0.0259
Epilepsy	0.0124	0.0379	0.0288	0.0290
Extremity amputation or loss	0.0125	0.0061	0.0171	0.0023
GYN condition	0.0027	0.0072	0.0019	0.0063
Genitourinary condition	0.0100	0.0195	0.0127	0.0191
Hemic condition	0.0030	0.0123	0.0048	0.0090
Infectious disease	0.0033	0.0072	0.0035	0.0095
Major depressive disorder	0.0355	0.0631	0.0301	0.0641
Muscle injury	0.0171	0.0253	0.0373	0.0324
Other code	0.0047	0.0145	0.0362	0.0088
Other mental disorder	0.0152	0.0282	0.0145	0.0476
Other musculoskeletal disease	0.0401	0.0457	0.0488	0.0457
Other musculoskeletal injury	0.1200	0.1333	0.2081	0.0900
Other neurological condition	0.1185	0.1541	0.1446	0.1541
Other respiratory condition	0.0167	0.0143	0.0106	0.0333
Other spinal injury	0.0276	0.0130	0.0180	0.0208
PTSD	0.1925	0.0678	0.1563	0.0623
Schizophrenia	0.0105	0.0262	0.0175	0.0163
Sense organ condition	0.0215	0.0238	0.0254	0.0215
Skin condition	0.0210	0.0147	0.0204	0.0132
Spinal injury 5237	0.0795	0.0743	0.0666	0.0281
Spinal injury 5241	0.0364	0.0410	0.0287	0.0343
Spinal injury 5242	0.0797	0.0154	0.0193	0.0377
Spinal injury 5243	0.0659	0.0308	0.0193	0.1244
Traumatic brain injury (TBI)	0.0582	0.0193	0.0895	0.0125

Table A.6
Disability Regression Coefficients, Standard Errors, and Marginal Effects: Multinomial Probit for Disability Disposition

Variable	PDRL			TDRL			Separation
	Estimate	Std. Error	Marg. Effect	Estimate	Std. Error	Marg. Effect	Marg. Effect
	Army and Navy DES						
FY07	—	—	—	—	—	—	—
FY08	0.0683	0.1420	0.0061	0.0485	0.0732	0.0043	–0.0104
FY09	0.8989	0.1280	0.1179	0.0478	0.0761	–0.0490	–0.0689
FY10	0.9389	0.1418	0.1455	–0.2991	0.0927	–0.1136	–0.0319
Age	0.0703	0.0020	0.0070	0.0377	0.0019	0.0022	–0.0093
Female	–0.1213	0.0375	–0.0166	0.0043	0.0318	0.0085	0.0081
Reserve component	–0.4138	0.1646	–0.0560	0.0053	0.1075	0.0274	0.0286
Officer	–0.0581	0.1681	–0.0124	0.0719	0.1687	0.0166	–0.0042
Married	–0.0111	0.0281	0.0020	–0.0552	0.0246	–0.0092	0.0071
IDES	0.2793	0.0369	0.0436	–0.0946	0.0360	–0.0348	–0.0088
Not deployed since 2001	—	—	—	—	—	—	—
Deployed within 1 year of MEB	0.3274	0.0357	0.0271	0.2650	0.0321	0.0264	–0.0535
Deployed within 1-2 years of MEB	0.3323	0.0370	0.0329	0.1851	0.0337	0.0118	–0.0447
Deployed within 2-3 years of MEB	0.2630	0.0497	0.0284	0.1095	0.0452	0.0027	–0.0311
Deployed within 3-4 years of MEB	0.2844	0.0626	0.0305	0.1213	0.0578	0.0035	–0.0340
Deployed 4+ years before MEB	0.3540	0.0610	0.0394	0.1283	0.0576	0.0003	–0.0397
Infantry, gun crews, seamanship	0.0708	0.0442	0.0083	0.0200	0.0387	–0.0010	–0.0073
Electronic equipment repairers	–0.0412	0.0648	–0.0093	0.0587	0.0532	0.0131	–0.0038
Communications, intelligence	0.0289	0.0555	0.0039	–0.0005	0.0495	–0.0019	–0.0020
Healthcare specialists	–0.0234	0.0611	–0.0077	0.0713	0.0533	0.0142	–0.0065
Other technical & allied specialists	0.0306	0.0857	–0.0043	0.1316	0.0764	0.0216	–0.0173
Functional support & administration	0.1479	0.0513	0.0132	0.1045	0.0453	0.0092	–0.0224
Electrical/mechanical equipment repairers	—	—	—	—	—	—	—
Craftsworkers	–0.1546	0.0800	–0.0160	–0.0743	0.0689	–0.0034	0.0194
Service and supply handlers	–0.0404	0.0479	–0.0053	–0.0016	0.0423	0.0023	0.0030
Non-occupational	0.1024	0.0896	–0.0160	0.4656	0.0635	0.0767	–0.0607
Tactical operations officers	0.6649	0.1722	0.0581	0.4897	0.1721	0.0450	–0.1031
Intelligence officers	1.0529	0.2911	0.0876	0.8445	0.2868	0.0836	–0.1712
Engineering & maintenance officers	0.9753	0.2095	0.1081	0.3620	0.2103	0.0023	–0.1104
Scientists and professionals	0.5566	0.3275	0.0572	0.2766	0.3194	0.0138	–0.0710
Healthcare officers	0.3403	0.2395	0.0079	0.5923	0.2289	0.0842	–0.0920

Table A.6—Continued

Variable	PDRL			TDRL			Separation
	Estimate	Std. Error	Marg. Effect	Estimate	Std. Error	Marg. Effect	Marg. Effect
Administrators	0.7102	0.2443	0.0568	0.6049	0.2400	0.0627	−0.1196
Supply, procurement officers	0.7074	0.2371	0.0647	0.4768	0.2353	0.0400	−0.1046
Non-occupational	0.8721	0.2422	0.0919	0.3976	0.2399	0.0153	−0.1072
DoD-unique musculoskeletal diseases	0.5247	0.0369	0.0517	0.2951	0.0341	0.0192	−0.0709
DoD-unique musculoskeletal Injuries	0.7326	0.0418	0.0526	0.7178	0.0358	0.0815	−0.1341
DOD-unique musculoskeletal injuries	0.1740	0.1078	0.0198	0.0571	0.0969	−0.0009	−0.0188
Anxiety disorder	1.3648	0.0893	0.0122	2.6771	0.0720	0.3914	−0.4037
Arthritis	—	—	—	—	—	—	—
Asthma	2.8947	0.0845	0.1857	3.1823	0.0745	0.3839	−0.5696
Bipolar disorder	2.4182	0.0887	0.1382	2.9240	0.0716	0.3682	−0.5063
Cardiovascular condition	2.2011	0.0819	0.1757	1.8808	0.0772	0.1955	−0.3712
Digestive condition	2.5723	0.0794	0.1810	2.5789	0.0701	0.2966	−0.4776
Endocrine condition	1.0544	0.0992	0.0796	0.9730	0.0844	0.1065	−0.1861
Epilepsy	2.2573	0.1044	0.1150	2.9471	0.0797	0.3826	−0.4976
Extremity amputation or loss	5.6417	0.2259	0.5497	3.2703	0.2342	0.2237	−0.7734
GYN condition	2.4881	0.2069	0.1801	2.4158	0.1849	0.2728	−0.4529
Genitourinary condition	2.6481	0.1212	0.1835	2.6991	0.1105	0.3132	−0.4967
Hemic condition	2.5981	0.2003	0.1435	3.2189	0.1699	0.4094	−0.5529
Infectious disease	2.9430	0.1978	0.2024	3.0233	0.1780	0.3523	−0.5547
Major depressive disorder	1.8315	0.0662	0.0774	2.6398	0.0561	0.3549	−0.4323
Muscle injury	2.2399	0.0846	0.2315	1.0922	0.0861	0.0519	−0.2834
Other code	1.2775	0.1465	0.1160	0.8731	0.1311	0.0744	−0.1904
Other mental disorder	1.8019	0.0938	0.0940	2.3190	0.0804	0.2994	−0.3934
Other musculoskeletal disease	1.0739	0.0610	0.0788	1.0257	0.0543	0.1147	−0.1935
Other musculoskeletal injury	1.4192	0.0391	0.1179	1.1416	0.0360	0.1133	−0.2312
Other neurological condition	2.1886	0.0400	0.1648	2.0253	0.0368	0.2221	−0.3869
Other respiratory condition	2.2453	0.0960	0.1586	2.2409	0.0900	0.2570	−0.4157
Other spinal injury	1.3627	0.0753	0.1299	0.8350	0.0766	0.0621	−0.1920
Schizophrenia	3.1759	0.1148	0.1845	3.7932	0.0972	0.4751	−0.6596
Sense organ condition	2.1298	0.0786	0.1927	1.4670	0.0791	0.1260	−0.3187
Skin condition	2.3524	0.0873	0.2072	1.7076	0.0880	0.1548	−0.3620
Spinal injury 5237	0.8638	0.0511	0.0807	0.5555	0.0473	0.0440	−0.1247
Spinal injury 5241	1.9266	0.0657	0.1602	1.5462	0.0630	0.1532	−0.3134
Spinal injury 5242	1.0261	0.0507	0.0923	0.7148	0.0540	0.0622	−0.1544

Table A.6—Continued

	PDRL			TDRL			Separation
Variable	Estimate	Std. Error	Marg. Effect	Estimate	Std. Error	Marg. Effect	Marg. Effect
Spinal injury 5243	1.1496	0.0545	0.0908	0.9983	0.0532	0.1049	−0.1957
Traumatic brain injury (TBI)	2.4958	0.0810	0.1677	2.6259	0.0761	0.3099	−0.4776
Army	0.2763	0.1109	0.1120	−1.1689	0.0609	−0.2268	0.1147
Marines	−0.0790	0.1538	−0.0083	−0.0371	0.0780	−0.0016	0.0098
Army_FY08	0.8038	0.1486	0.0831	0.3909	0.0821	0.0184	−0.1016
Army_FY09	0.4509	0.1342	0.0331	0.4310	0.0845	0.0482	−0.0813
Army_FY10	0.6117	0.1482	0.0476	0.5419	0.1024	0.0578	−0.1054
Marines_FY08	−0.1581	0.2087	−0.0108	−0.1636	0.1048	−0.0191	0.0299
Marines_FY09	−0.0315	0.1828	0.0099	−0.2202	0.1070	−0.0374	0.0275
Marines_FY10	0.0405	0.2012	0.0229	−0.2725	0.1304	−0.0513	0.0284
Army_Reserve	0.3354	0.1674	0.0446	0.0086	0.1121	−0.0199	−0.0246
Marine_Reserve	0.4467	0.2165	0.0529	0.1129	0.1410	−0.0084	−0.0445
Constant	−6.2734	0.1263		−2.9463	0.0802		
		Air Force DES					
FY09	—	—	—	—	—	—	—
FY10	0.2359	0.0779	0.0341	0.0884	0.0716	−0.0021	−0.0321
Age	0.1496	0.0059	0.0235	0.0360	0.0057	−0.0058	−0.0177
Female	−0.1315	0.0831	−0.0123	−0.1225	0.0755	−0.0152	0.0275
Reserve component	−1.1459	0.1312	−0.1817	−0.2576	0.1279	0.0484	0.1334
IDES	0.2103	0.1331	0.0234	0.1554	0.1288	0.0152	−0.0386
Not deployed since 2001	—	—	—	—	—	—	—
Deployed within 1 year of MEB	−0.0446	0.1557	−0.0399	0.3448	0.1329	0.0811	−0.0412
Deployed within 1–2 years of MEB	0.1392	0.1165	0.0026	0.2417	0.1093	0.0411	−0.0437
Deployed within 2–3 years of MEB	0.1687	0.1375	−0.0005	0.3335	0.1299	0.0588	−0.0583
VASRD1	−0.2966	0.1582	−0.0118	−0.4475	0.1569	−0.0725	0.0843
VASRD2	0.3490	0.1120	0.0728	−0.1109	0.1125	−0.0570	−0.0158
VASRD3	0.2031	0.1069	0.0290	0.0808	0.1045	−0.0007	−0.0282
VASRD4	1.2268	0.0947	0.1280	0.9956	0.0910	0.1089	−0.2369
VASRD5	0.8792	0.1220	0.0348	1.3304	0.1112	0.2157	−0.2505
VASRD6	1.4983	0.1260	0.0567	2.2954	0.1133	0.3739	−0.4305
VASRD7	2.4214	0.4706	0.2029	2.5045	0.4603	0.3353	−0.5382
VASRD8	0.7265	0.6016	−0.1514	3.0496	0.3291	0.6135	−0.4621
Constant	−5.8845	0.2098	—	−2.3174	0.1875	—	—
	−5.9449	0.2113	—	−2.3405	0.1881	—	—

Table A.7
Disability Regression Coefficients, Standard Errors, and Marginal Effects: Ordinary Least Squares for Disability Rating (Army and Navy DES)

	Army/Navy/Marine Corps		Air Force	
Variable	**Estimate**	**Std. Error**	**Estimate**	**Std. Error**
Intercept	−0.6864	0.5621	−0.9094	1.6060
FY07	—	—	—	—
FY08	1.2034	0.5816	—	—
FY09	4.3560	0.5979	—	—
FY10	2.5439	0.7349	0.6192	0.6203
Age	0.3923	0.0120	0.5865	0.0485
Female	−0.6439	0.2165	−1.9090	0.7095
Reserve component	−2.2827	0.7818	−1.1972	1.0122
Officer	2.3172	1.0374	19.4089	6.7029
Married	−0.3250	0.1613	0.9286	0.6468
IDES	3.0440	0.2295	2.5311	1.0694
Not deployed since 2001	—	—	—	—
Deployed within 1 year of MEB	2.0712	0.2133	3.7478	1.1648
Deployed within 1–2 years of MEB	2.5057	0.2202	2.2132	0.9555
Deployed within 2–3 years of MEB	2.3477	0.2852	3.1761	1.1164
Deployed within 3–4 years of MEB	2.6965	0.3637	1.4780	1.3348
Deployed 4+ years before MEB	3.5691	0.3726	−0.0108	0.9589
Infantry, gun crews, seamanship	0.5119	0.2536	1.1228	1.2464
Electronic equipment repairers	−0.7140	0.3729	0.8790	1.4201
Communications, intelligence	−0.1143	0.3207	1.0110	1.2956
Healthcare specialists	−0.1526	0.3465	1.9585	1.2849
Other technical & allied specialists	0.1853	0.5077	1.5090	1.6246
Functional support & administration	0.7205	0.3062	0.3027	1.0159
Electrical/mechanical equipment repairers	—	—	—	—
Craftsworkers	−0.5402	0.4523	−1.0176	1.6575
Service and supply handlers	−0.3272	0.2789	1.2406	1.1407
Non-occupational	1.0223	0.4607	3.8829	1.4793
Tactical operations officers	3.8973	1.0717	−10.4897	7.0787
Intelligence officers	3.0416	1.7640	−22.8975	8.1521
Engineering & maintenance officers	3.4743	1.2990	−22.9164	7.7188
Scientists and professionals	3.9836	1.8883	−14.3323	7.6382
Healthcare officers	2.5643	1.4386	−23.2809	6.9915
Administrators	2.2599	1.5241	−22.4420	7.5264
Supply, procurement officers	3.1510	1.4274	−18.2877	7.4702
Non-occupational	1.9850	1.4960	0.0000	—
DoD-unique musculoskeletal diseases	2.7980	0.2026	−4.1228	1.6371
DoD-unique musculoskeletal Injuries	5.3376	0.2342	−0.7020	1.9297
DOD-unique muscle injuries	1.4937	0.6020	−4.6367	3.8802
Anxiety disorder	19.0332	0.5190	12.7093	2.2991

Table A.7—Continued

	Army/Navy/Marine Corps		Air Force	
Variable	**Estimate**	**Std. Error**	**Estimate**	**Std. Error**
Arthritis	—	—	—	—
Asthma	16.3448	0.5099	11.1941	1.1746
Bipolar disorder	20.4474	0.5525	18.7515	1.6896
Cardiovascular condition	19.3697	0.5454	9.8119	1.5524
Digestive condition	18.7556	0.4874	14.8842	1.4937
Endocrine condition	9.5724	0.5933	7.1299	1.9594
Epilepsy	24.0452	0.5731	12.6329	1.7617
Extremity amputation or loss	45.5512	0.6751	43.7874	5.0620
GYN condition	22.4843	1.3250	43.6531	3.9091
Genitourinary condition	28.8115	0.7005	22.5656	2.3431
Hemic condition	48.5816	1.1328	47.2783	3.2760
Infectious disease	29.7572	1.2076	23.1786	2.7889
Major depressive disorder	19.6434	0.3958	15.5913	1.2930
Muscle injury	12.6339	0.5321	6.4930	1.9058
Other code	8.0315	0.7737	30.4467	4.0169
Other mental disorder	16.5536	0.5810	10.9048	1.4863
Other musculoskeletal disease	8.1932	0.3753	11.5344	1.3853
Other musculoskeletal injury	8.4176	0.2310	3.1300	1.1259
Other neurological condition	15.5842	0.2293	15.9882	0.9187
Other respiratory condition	21.7527	0.5962	16.3657	1.7882
Other spinal injury	9.3991	0.4774	4.2638	2.0633
Schizophrenia	31.0517	0.6606	32.6511	2.5229
Sense organ condition	11.3477	0.5045	7.5000	2.1757
Skin condition	17.9723	0.5267	17.7950	2.5406
Spinal injury 5237	5.3354	0.2845	3.4256	1.8740
Spinal injury 5241	10.4828	0.4081	6.3168	2.0189
Spinal injury 5242	5.8141	0.3144	2.5863	1.3507
Spinal injury 5243	6.8913	0.3292	4.2260	1.0943
Traumatic brain injury (TBI)	21.5484	0.3329	23.1047	2.1922
PTSD	28.9561	0.2224	30.8155	1.2382
Army	-6.7098	0.4660	—	—
Marine Corps	-3.2132	0.6043	—	—
Army x FY08	6.5755	0.6272	—	—
Army x FY09	6.7694	0.6391	—	—
Army x FY10	8.9994	0.7790	—	—
Marine Corps x FY08	1.1986	0.8038	—	—
Marine Corps x FY09	1.4839	0.8161	—	—
Marine Corps x FY10	1.9238	0.9969	—	—
Army x Reserve	2.6248	0.8030	—	—
Marine Corps x Reserve	2.5707	1.0146	—	—

Table A.8
Disability Regression Coefficients, Standard Errors, and Marginal Effects: OLS for (Log) DES Processing Time

Variable	Army		Navy/Marine Corps	
	Estimate	Std. Error	Estimate	Std.Error
Army and Navy MEB Processing Time				
Intercept	4.2091	0.0232	3.7147	0.0415
FY07	—	—	—	—
FY08	0.1347	0.0103	0.1151	0.0167
FY09	0.0209	0.0107	0.1302	0.0192
FY10	0.0169	0.0132	0.0731	0.0236
Age	0.0052	0.0006	−0.0020	0.0013
Female	−0.0058	0.0109	−0.0156	0.0183
Reserve component	−0.0461	0.0117	0.0536	0.0234
Officer	0.0279	0.0509	−0.0155	0.1482
Married	0.0467	0.0080	0.0328	0.0137
IDES	0.3656	0.0143	−0.0227	0.0266
Deployed within 1 year of MEB	0.0684	0.0106	0.0420	0.0215
Deployed within 1–2 years of MEB	0.0487	0.0112	0.0258	0.0197
Deployed within 2–3 years of MEB	0.0109	0.0145	0.0153	0.0237
Deployed within 3–4 years of MEB	0.0333	0.0185	0.0477	0.0305
Deployed 4+ years before MEB	0.0305	0.0204	−0.0069	0.0278
Infantry, gun crews, seamanship	0.0045	0.0129	−0.0037	0.0206
Electronic equipment repairers	0.0160	0.0202	0.0209	0.0257
Communications, intelligence	−0.0215	0.0157	0.0332	0.0301
Healthcare specialists	−0.0384	0.0174	0.0352	0.0349
Other technical & allied specialists	−0.0640	0.0245	0.0026	0.0551
Functional support & administration	0.0360	0.0156	0.0496	0.0246
Electrical/mechanical equipment repairers	—	—	—	—
Craftsworkers	0.0276	0.0233	0.0324	0.0349
Service and supply handlers	−0.0035	0.0139	0.0611	0.0254
Non-occupational	−0.0672	0.0312	−0.1697	0.0281
Tactical operations officers	−0.1723	0.0515	−0.0259	0.1617
Intelligence officers	−0.0755	0.0875	−0.3905	0.2138
Engineering & maintenance officers	−0.0609	0.0672	−0.0354	0.1608
Scientists and professionals	0.0431	0.1034	0.2239	0.2009
Healthcare officers	−0.1186	0.0719	0.0801	0.1740
Administrators	−0.0230	0.0789	−0.2679	0.1931
Supply, procurement officers	0.0939	0.0709	−0.1255	0.1744
Non-occupational	−0.0478	0.0763	−0.0876	0.1769

Table A.8—Continued

	Army		Navy/Marine Corps	
Variable	**Estimate**	**Std. Error**	**Estimate**	**Std.Error**
DoD-unique musculoskeletal diseases	0.0518	0.0096	0.0856	0.0225
DoD-unique musculoskeletal Injuries	0.0555	0.0116	0.0515	0.0210
DOD-unique muscle injuries	0.0012	0.0292	−0.0124	0.0670
Anxiety disorder	0.2903	0.0244	0.1106	0.0618
Arthritis	0.1595	0.0236	0.0926	0.0535
Asthma	—	—	—	—
Bipolar disorder	0.2236	0.0304	0.0566	0.0373
Cardiovascular condition	0.1354	0.0287	0.0643	0.0471
Digestive condition	0.1410	0.0268	0.0856	0.0337
Endocrine condition	0.1718	0.0314	0.0467	0.0492
Epilepsy	0.2415	0.0329	0.1170	0.0383
Extremity amputation or loss	0.1483	0.0337	0.0623	0.0652
GYN condition	0.0560	0.0717	0.0509	0.0952
Genitourinary condition	0.0520	0.0369	0.0551	0.0512
Hemic condition	0.1541	0.0694	0.0879	0.0677
Infectious disease	0.1889	0.0658	0.0059	0.0916
Major depressive disorder	0.2849	0.0204	0.1226	0.0326
Muscle injury	0.0641	0.0281	0.0473	0.0501
Other code	0.2754	0.0540	0.0225	0.0466
Other mental disorder	0.2873	0.0303	0.1244	0.0458
Other musculoskeletal disease	0.1020	0.0190	0.1883	0.0367
Other musculoskeletal injury	0.0936	0.0118	0.0012	0.0202
Other neurological condition	0.1314	0.0118	0.0961	0.0196
Other respiratory condition	0.1664	0.0295	0.1493	0.0629
Other spinal injury	0.1422	0.0225	0.2184	0.0551
Schizophrenia	0.1689	0.0359	0.1095	0.0452
Sense organ condition	0.1355	0.0256	0.0856	0.0420
Skin condition	0.1192	0.0260	0.0148	0.0530
Spinal injury 5237	0.1512	0.0142	0.0801	0.0264
Spinal injury 5241	0.1272	0.0211	0.0034	0.0352
Spinal injury 5242	0.1780	0.0144	0.0055	0.0666
Spinal injury 5243	0.1363	0.0155	0.1209	0.0435
Traumatic brain injury (TBI)	0.2637	0.0159	0.3215	0.0352
PTSD	0.3061	0.0107	0.1458	0.0242

Table A.8—Continued

Variable	Army		Navy/Marine Corps	
	Estimate	Std. Error	Estimate	Std.Error
Army and Navy PEB Processing Time				
Intercept	3.6215	0.0171	2.9419	0.0312
FY07	—	—	—	—
FY08	0.2307	0.0085	0.2690	0.0134
FY09	0.2465	0.0087	0.5002	0.0150
FY10	0.2218	0.0105	0.5289	0.0182
Age	0.0102	0.0005	0.0103	0.0010
Female	0.0085	0.0090	0.0010	0.0150
Reserve component	−0.1691	0.0091	0.1212	0.0186
Officer	0.0074	0.0430	0.0970	0.1226
Married	0.0966	0.0067	0.0059	0.0113
IDES	0.2096	0.0103	0.0043	0.0177
Not deployed since 2001	0.1717	0.0086	0.0325	0.0175
Deployed within 1 year of MEB	—	—	—	—
Deployed within 1–2 years of MEB	0.2060	0.0092	0.0401	0.0161
Deployed within 2–3 years of MEB	0.1963	0.0121	0.0493	0.0196
Deployed within 3–4 years of MEB	0.1843	0.0155	0.0876	0.0252
Deployed 4+ years before MEB	0.1584	0.0172	0.0005	0.0229
Infantry, gun crews, Seamanship	−0.0237	0.0107	−0.0393	0.0165
Electronic equipment repairers	−0.0602	0.0167	0.0092	0.0212
Communications, intelligence	−0.0311	0.0131	−0.0128	0.0247
Healthcare specialists	−0.1398	0.0141	0.0016	0.0287
Other technical & allied specialists	−0.0511	0.0204	0.0512	0.0454
Functional support & administration	0.0700	0.0130	0.0148	0.0201
Electrical/mechanical equipment repairers	—	—	—	—
Craftsworkers	−0.0219	0.0195	−0.0140	0.0285
Service and supply handlers	−0.0264	0.0115	0.0089	0.0208
Non-occupational	−0.1522	0.0258	−0.2384	0.0207
Tactical operations officers	0.0409	0.0435	−0.0145	0.1338
Intelligence officers	0.0550	0.0746	0.3209	0.1769
Engineering & maintenance officers	0.0394	0.0560	0.0548	0.1332
Scientists and professionals	0.1098	0.0889	−0.1227	0.1659
Health care officers	0.1401	0.0607	0.0964	0.1439
Administrators	0.1693	0.0672	−0.1410	0.1598
Supply, procurement officers	0.1256	0.0594	0.0314	0.1443
Non-occupational	0.0478	0.0643	0.0505	0.1440
DoD-unique musculoskeletal diseases	−0.0176	0.0079	0.0553	0.0185
DoD-unique musculoskeletal injuries	−0.0361	0.0095	0.0417	0.0174

Table A.8—Continued

	Army		Navy/Marine Corps	
Variable	**Estimate**	**Std. Error**	**Estimate**	**Std.Error**
DOD-unique muscle injuries	0.0379	0.0242	−0.0364	0.0554
Anxiety disorder	0.1577	0.0203	0.0636	0.0511
Arthritis	0.1673	0.0196	0.0734	0.0442
Asthma	—	—	—	—
Bipolar disorder	0.2411	0.0256	0.0819	0.0308
Cardiovascular condition	0.1603	0.0241	0.1629	0.0390
Digestive condition	0.1229	0.0224	0.0079	0.0279
Endocrine condition	0.1272	0.0264	0.0709	0.0406
Epilepsy	0.2486	0.0277	0.0811	0.0315
Extremity amputation or loss	0.0905	0.0272	0.2061	0.0527
GYN condition	0.1823	0.0612	−0.1268	0.0788
Genitourinary condition	0.1300	0.0310	0.0581	0.0423
Hemic condition	0.1958	0.0582	0.0292	0.0559
Infectious disease	0.1867	0.0551	0.1127	0.0758
Major depressive disorder	0.1545	0.0172	0.1078	0.0269
Muscle injury	0.1793	0.0234	0.0523	0.0415
Other code	0.2401	0.0454	−0.0875	0.0384
Other mental disorder	0.1653	0.0253	0.1622	0.0379
Other musculoskeletal disease	−0.0055	0.0158	0.1347	0.0303
Other musculoskeletal injury	0.0386	0.0099	−0.0184	0.0166
Other neurological condition	0.1369	0.0099	0.0768	0.0162
Other respiratory condition	0.1356	0.0248	0.0131	0.0520
Other spinal injury	0.0868	0.0190	0.0972	0.0455
Schizophrenia	0.1932	0.0299	0.1196	0.0372
Sense organ condition	0.1432	0.0215	0.1212	0.0347
Skin condition	0.1633	0.0216	0.1761	0.0433
Spinal injury 5237	0.1296	0.0117	0.0897	0.0218
Spinal injury 5241	0.0910	0.0176	0.0540	0.0290
Spinal injury 5242	0.0505	0.0121	0.1363	0.0551
Spinal injury 5243	0.0302	0.0129	0.1531	0.0360
Traumatic brain injury (TBI)	0.0948	0.0133	0.2201	0.0289
PTSD	0.1117	0.0089	0.1159	0.0199

Bibliography

Abraham, J. M., and R. Feldman, "Taking Up or Turning Down: New Estimates of Household Demand for Employer-Sponsored Health Insurance," *Inquiry*, Vol. 47, Spring 2010, pp. 17–32.

Adamson, David M., M. Audrey Burnam, Rachel M. Burns, Leah B. Caldarone, Robert A. Cox, Elizabeth D'Amico, Claudia Diaz, Christine Eibner, Gail Fisher, Todd C. Helmus, Terri Tanielian, Benjamin R. Karney, Beau Kilmer, Grant N. Marshall, Laurie T. Martin, Lisa S. Meredith, Karen N. Metscher, Karen Chan Osilla, Rosalie Liccardo Pacula, Rajeev Ramchand, Jeanne S. Ringel, Terry L. Schell, Jerry M. Sollinger, Lisa H. Jaycox, Mary E. Vaiana, Kayla M. Williams, and Michael R. Yochelson, *Invisible Wounds of War: Psychological and Cognitive Injuries, Their Consequences, and Services to Assist Recovery*, Santa Monica, Calif.: RAND Corporation, 2008. As of July 23, 2011: http://www.rand.org/pubs/monographs/MG720.html

Bansak, Cynthia, and Steven Raphael, "The State Children's Health Insurance Program and Job Mobility: Identifying Job Lock among Working Parents in Near-Poor Households," *Industrial and Labor Relations Review*, Vol. 61, No. 4, 2008, pp. 564–579.

Brauner, Marygail K., Timothy Jackson, and Elizabeth K. Gayton, *Medical Readiness of the Reserve Component*, Santa Monica, Calif.: RAND Corporation, 2012. As of April 16, 2012: http://www.rand.org/pubs/monographs/MG1105.html

Brook, R. H., J. E. Ware, Jr., W. H. Rogers, E. B. Keeler, A. R. Davies, C. A. Donald, G. A. Goldberg, K. N. Lohr, P. C. Masthay, and J. P. Newhouse, "Does Free Care Improve Adults' Health?—Results from a Randomized Controlled Trial," *The New England Journal of Medicine*, Vol. 309, No. 23, 1983, pp. 1426–1434.

Chandra, Amitabh, Jonathan Gruber, and Robin McKnight, "The Importance of the Individual Mandate—Evidence from Massachusetts," *New England Journal of Medicine*, Vol. 36, No. 44, January 27, 2011, pp. 293–295.

Christensen, Eric, Joyce McMahon, Elizabeth Schaefer, Ted Jaditz, and Dan Harris, *Final Report for the Veterans' Disability Benefits Commission: Compensation, Survey Results,and Selected Topics*: Alexandria, Va.: Center for Naval Analysis, 2007.

The Commonwealth Fund, "Health Reform Resource Center: What's in the Affordable Care Act?" 2011. As of May 23, 2011: http://www.commonwealthfund.org/Health-Reform/Health-Reform-Resource.aspx

Defense Manpower Data Center, *November 2008 Status of Forces Survey of Reserve Component Members: Administration, Datasets, and Codebook*, DMDC Report No. 2009-024, 2009.

Department of Defense, *Comprehensive Review of the Future Role of the Reserve Component:* Volume I, *Executive Summary & Main Report*, 2011.

Ellis, Randall P., and Ching-To Albert Ma, "Health Insurance, Cost Expectations, and Adverse Job Turnover," *Health Economics,* Vol. 20, No. 1, 2011, pp. 27–44.

Finkelstein, Amy, Sarah Taubman, Bill Wright, Mira Bernstein, Jonathan Gruber, Joseph P. Newhouse, Heidi Allen, and Katherine Baicker, "The Oregon Health Insurance Experiment: Evidence from the First Year," Cambridge, Mass.: National Bureau of Economic Research, NBER Working Paper, 2011.

Freeman, Joseph D., Srikanth Kadiyala, Janice F. Bell, and Diane P. Martin, "The Causal Effect of Health Insurance on Utilization and Outcomes in Adults: A Systematic Review of US Studies," *Medical Care,* Vol. 46, No. 10, 2008, pp. 1023–1032.

Girosi, Federico, Amado Cordova, Christine Eibner, Carole Roan Gresenz, Emmett B. Keeler, Jeanne S. Ringel, Jeffrey Sullivan, John Bertko, Melinda Beeuwkes Buntin, and Raffaele Vardavas, *Overview of the Compare Microsimulation Model,* Santa Monica, Calif.: RAND Corporation, WR-650, 2009. As of June 7, 2011:
http://www.rand.org/pubs/working_papers/WR650.html

Government Accountability Office, *Military and Veterans Disability System: Pilot Has Achieved Some Goals, but Further Planning and Monitoring Needed,* GAO 11-633T, 2010.

———, *Military and Veterans Disability System: Worldwide Deployment of Integrated System Warrants Careful Monitoring,* GAO-11-633T, 2011.

———, *Military Disability Retirement: Closer Monitoring Would Improve the Temporary Retirement Process,* GAO 09-239, 2009.

———, *Military Disability System: Improved Oversight Needed to Ensure Consistent and Timely Outcomes for Reserve and Active Duty Service Members,* GAO 06-362, 2006.

———, *Military Health Care: Cost Data Indicate That Tricare Reserve Select Premiums Exceeded the Costs of Providing Program Benefits,* GAO-08-104, 2007.

Gruber, J., and K. Simon, "Crowd-Out 10 Years Later: Have Recent Public Insurance Expansions Crowded Out Private Health Insurance?" *Journal of Health Economics,* Vol. 27, February 2008, pp. 201–211.

Gruber, Jonathan, "Covering the Uninsured in the United States," *Journal of Economic Literature,* Vol. 46, No. 3, September 2008, pp. 571–606.

Gruber, Jonathan, and Brigitte C. Madrian, "Health Insurance, Labor Supply, and Job Mobility: A Critical Review of the Literature," Cambridge, Mass.: National Bureau of Economic Research, NBER Working Paper, 2002.

Hosek, Susan, "Tricare Reserve Select: Would Extending Eligibility to All Reservists Be Cost Effective?" in *The New Guard and Reserve,* John D. Winkler and Barbara A. Bicksler (eds.), San Ramon, Calif.: Falcon Books, 2010.

Institute of Medicine, *America's Uninsured Crisis: Consequences for Health and Health Care,* 2009.

Kaiser Family Foundation and Health Research and Educational Trust, *Employer Health Benefits: 2010 Annual Survey,* 2010.

Levy, Helen, and David Meltzer, "The Impact of Health Insurance on Health," *Annual Review of Public Health,* Vol. 29, 2008, pp. 399–409.

Mariano, Louis T., Sheila N. Kirby, Christine Eibner, and Scott Naftel, *Civilian Health Insurance Options of Military Retirees: Findings from a Pilot Survey,* Santa Monica, Calif.: RAND Corporation,